I0429391

NatMed4u.com
A View on Cancer

Natural Medicine in Cancer Treatment & Prevention

Ronald Fisher, ND

Caryn Wichmann, ND

Copyright © 2011 Ronald J Fisher, ND & Caryn H Wichmann, ND, Perpetual
Wellbeing Pty Ltd, Australia

All rights reserved.

ISBN- 10: 1466410647
ISBN-13: 978-1466410640

DEDICATION

This book is dedicated to those many clients who have courageously confronted the issues surrounding cancer. They have taught and inspired us to constantly pursue the underlying causes of cancer.

CONTENTS

ACKNOWLEDGMENTS

We acknowledge the outstanding work by many groups of scientists and researchers around the world who make the results of their research freely available through internet publications. Without the availability of this work we could not provide a high level service to our clients and this book would not be possible.

We are grateful for the dedicated work of our fellow Australians who work in the area of natural medicine and willingly support us with ideas and research. In particular, we acknowledge the extensive work of Henry Osiecki, Janet Schloss, and Kerry Bone who have provided outstanding leadership in finding ways that natural medicine can assist people to 'live with cancer'.

1   INTRODUCTION

About 33,000 people worldwide every day of the year receive the diagnosis from their doctor that 'you have cancer'. The prognosis and treatment options are then outlined for you and quite often you are recommended for urgent surgery, chemotherapy and, or radiation therapy. Sometimes the issue is less urgent and you are put on a 'wait and watch' list. While others are informed that there are no treatment options, and they should go home and get their will into order and make the most of the few months they have left.

No matter what you are told in this meeting with your medical practitioner, there is another action that you can take. You can decide to get as healthy as possible. A few informed doctors will tell you about this action but most have not studied the science of 'getting healthy' – they have studied the science of medical cures for illnesses. The natural medicine solutions that we outline in this book are all about supporting this process of getting healthy.

The knowledge and skills that the doctors, oncologists and surgeons have is highly developed and their recommendations will invariably be good ones. If you are not convinced that they are giving you good advice then you can always get a second opinion from another qualified medical practitioner.

It is not recommended that you 'get healthy' or use natural medicines instead of undergoing a medical procedure – the medical procedures will invariably be your best chance of a cure – the getting healthy decision is all about improving the medical outcomes and improving your quality of life. Even if you have been told that you have only months to live and there are no medical actions to take – the 'getting healthy' action will still have lots of benefits for you. The reasons why we believe this, are outlined in this book.

The process of 'getting healthy' needs to be fitted in around the actions and advice of your medical practitioners. Consequently, in this book, we give you all the technical references about the natural medicines you can use, so that you are well positioned to check with your doctors that the actions you are taking will not conflict with any of the medical procedures and will usually compliment and make the medical procedures more effective.

The medical term for cancer is a malignant neoplasm. Cancer is actually a large group of diseases in which the malignant cells display uncontrolled growth, invasion that intrudes upon and destroys adjacent tissues, and often metastasizes, wherein the tumour cells spread to other locations in the body via the lymphatic system or through the bloodstream.

Research[1] published in 2008 indicated that on an annual basis more than 1 million Americans and more than 10 million people worldwide are expected to be diagnosed with cancer. The researchers found that only 5-10% of all cancer cases can be attributed to genetic defects, whereas the remaining 90-95% have their roots in the environment and lifestyle. The whole basis of natural medicine is to look for the underlying causes of illness. There are many obvious environmental causes of cancer including smoking, obesity, infection and radiation. However, the cause is often complicated by a number of issues working together. After all, not everyone who smokes, gets fat, has an infection or is exposed to radiation actually gets cancer.

Cell reproduction is an extremely complex process that is normally tightly regulated by several classes of genes, including oncogenes and tumour suppressor genes. The natural medicine approach to cancer is to put your body in a position where these regulatory processes can work properly. Even for the small percentage of people who have cancer linked to a genetic factor, there are benefits to be gained from a natural medicine approach where you focus on getting your genes to function normally.

Our focus throughout this book is to provide you with immediately usable information and to point you in the direction of where to focus your research efforts and what research to monitor.

References

1. Anand P, Kunnumakkara AB, Kunnumakara AB, et al, 2008, Cancer is a preventable disease that requires major lifestyle changes, *Pharm. Res*, 25 (9): 2097–116, PMC 2515569, PMID, 18626751.

2 WHAT DOES IT MEAN TO BE HEALTHY?

Really being healthy requires a lot more than 'feeling healthy'.

Before assessing whether you are healthy you need to understand one of the most important mechanisms that we have in our body, called 'Homeostasis'.

Homeostasis is the condition of equilibrium or balance in the body's internal environment, due to the ceaseless interplay of the body's many regulatory processes. Every structure in the body, from the cellular level to overall body systems, contribute in some way to keeping the internal environment of the body within normal limits. As an example of one of the many things monitored is blood glucose levels, which is maintained between 70 and 110 milligrams of glucose per 100 millilitres of blood.

To protect the internal environment, the body will detect undesirable substances entering the skin, nose or gastrointestinal system and mount a defence. Most often the immune system, nervous system and the endocrine system, working together or independently, provide the needed corrective measures. Our modern chemical filled environment makes constant demands on these systems, which means that to be healthy we need to maintain these systems in extremely good working order if we are going to remain healthy. A failure of our defence mechanisms is often an underlying cause of cancer.

A big issue with cancer patients is to appreciate that you have a lot more wrong with you than just cancer. If we put on a few extra kilograms, then our body makes the corrective actions to make our heart pump faster, etc to keep things in balance. Being fatter becomes the new normal and you are not consciously aware of the decline in your health. However, there are signs and symptoms that can alert you to underlying health problems. The skin and fat tissues are often used as temporary storage places for dangerous chemicals, until our liver or kidneys can assemble the required enzymes, or other proteins to deal with the offending substance. In some people they become 'time bombs' just waiting to go off. Unwanted appearance of lumps, bumps and other things on our skin can be a reflection of both poor management of our skin and poor management of our internal environment.

Because the mechanism of homeostasis works constantly, we have the feeling most of the time that 'we feel OK/ we feel comfortable', and even a person hugely overweight and clearly unhealthy will be maintained with this feeling of being OK. This is what we call the 'homeostasis melancholy' – your own body by its steady adaption process fools you into the very sad state of thinking that this is your new normal – that there is no need for change – when clearly there is. Frequently, the first time that you become aware that you have cancer is when you hear the words from the doctor. This is the biggest issue to address with anyone suffering from cancer. You have much more wrong with you than just cancer. You have an imbalance in many of your body systems that have resulted in them failing to protect you from cancer. You need to make changes to 'get healthy'.

Thus the feeling of 'being healthy' is not a good measure of whether you are actually healthy. Blood tests can indicate that you are out of balance in a particular area but the job of homeostasis is to keep things in balance so blood tests are only going to provide information after things have got dramatically out of control. Later in this book we will provide you with a checklist of symptoms which will give you an earlier warning sign than blood tests that things are going wrong. A healthy person always has plenty of energy to make the most of life.

3 THE 'GETTING HEALTHY' CHECKLIST

The following is a list of actions you can take to get healthy and live with cancer:

1. For many of the actions in this checklist you may need the help of someone qualified in nutritional medicine so they can help you obtain the most appropriate nutritional supplement or herbal medicine and work out the most appropriate dosages for you.

2. Remember that all cancers are not the same and scientific information is continually improving – so you will need to research (or get help researching) all the information provided here to see if it now applies to your cancer.

3. Eat healthy and avoid foods that feed cancer and create inflammation – see the chapters on this for more details.

4. Assess for nutrient deficiencies – see our chapter on this.

5. Monitor Your Symptoms – it is important that you monitor your progress and have some measurements to discuss issues with your doctor.

6. Avoid fad cures. 'Cures' sold on the internet or provided by non medical practitioners are highly unlikely to work and may actually make your condition worse – let your doctors work on the cures while you work on getting healthy.

7. Tone down your objectives. If the medical profession says that your malignant tumour cannot be removed or completely eradicated – accept this as the new reality and make your objective to be healthy and allow your body to manage the tumour so that you are effectively 'living with cancer'. The concept of trying to kill every cancer with external assistance may actually be counterproductive and it may be better to get your body healthy enough so that your body can manage the situation.

8. Avoid all environmental toxins. You need your liver to be working with the rest of your body to clear the cancer – environmental toxins will mean that your liver is hard at work getting rid of these – see our chapter on environmental toxins.

9. Exercise in moderate amounts to a level appropriate for your cancer – check with your doctor as to whether he/she recommends any restriction on exercise.

10. Gain control of your life and manage stress – see our chapter on this.

11. Express your emotions – it is OK to be 'pissed off' that you have cancer – be positive when you feel positive.

12. See if one of the mind body medicine techniques helps you. If not, don't persist – so check out psychotherapy, support groups, meditation, imagery, hypnosis, biofeedback, yoga, dance therapy, music and art therapies, prayer and mental healing – none of these will work in isolation but they can be a great support to other treatments – particularly meditation to relax the brain and then using a mental image of you getting healthier and your cancer reducing.

13. Check for drug and nutrient interactions. When preparing a treatment plan we first look at the drugs that the client is already taking. Quite often we find the drug list is extensive and hasn't been reviewed for interactions between the drugs. Bringing the interactions to the attention of one of the primary care physicians involved is the best way to rationalise the list and usually reduce many of the side effects arising from the drugs. To find out the interactions between

drugs a good starting point is the documentation supplied by the drug company with the drug (or information on the drug company website if you don't have the documentation). There are also a number of good websites run by doctors that provide information about drugs and their side effects. Later on, when you have developed your potential list of nutrients or herbs to take, it is then necessary to go back to the drug list and then compare each nutrient or herb with each of the drugs and any combined actions – this often results in many of the nutrients being taken off the list. Occasionally, if the oncologist is co-operative, the dose of some of the drugs can be reduced based on the known potentiating actions of the nutrients or herbs so you then get the anticancer benefits of the nutrients or herbs and the drug side effects are reduced. To achieve this you will usually need copies of the scientific references to supply to the oncologist as they often do not specialise in adding nutrients to their treatments.

14. Check for excessive toxic substances in the body such as copper and iron, as these can continue to restimulate the cancer as fast as the treatments reduce the cancer. If there are excessive levels it may be necessary to use a chelating agent – but be careful because, strangely enough, extremely low levels of trace elements (i.e. a deficiency) can also stimulate the cancer process. Iron chelators may be effective anti-tumour agents in some cancers – ovarian, lymphoma, myeloma and bladder cancer.

15. Protein absorption supplements – failing to absorb protein properly is common – we recommend supplements that support protein absorption to all cancer patients, as invariably the processes for protein absorption have been compromised.

16. Digestive Enzymes (Proteolytic enzymes) – in addition to being one of the ways of supporting protein absorption, these can also be effective in some cases for gradual breakdown of the tumour – read our chapter on these carefully before using them.

17. Fish Oils – these can usually help most cancer patients, but read our chapter on these before using them.

18. CoEnzymeQ10 – this has the potential to reduce tumour growth, stimulate the immune system and improve cellular energetics and so is a strong candidate to include in any cancer treatment unless it has negative interactions with the drugs being taken. Read our chapter on these before taking them as a supplement.

19. Assess for viral and bacterial issues – see our chapter on this.

20. Use additional nutritional and herbal supplements that will support your specific condition. When compiling this list we usually find 5 to 8 items that will specifically assist the body regain its normal control over the cancer. In the chapter on 'Other natural supplements to add to your cancer treatment' we have outlined the issues in regard to Resveratrol, Vitamin B6 (Pyridoxine, Selenium, Quercetin, Curcumin, Bromelain, Glutathione, Genistein, Vitamin D3 (cholecalciferol), Vitamin E, Vitamin C, Indole-3-carbinol, Lycopene, Green tea, Beetroot, Limonene, Boswellia serrata, and Baicalein.

4 GAINING CONTROL OF YOUR LIFE & MANAGING STRESS

Summary

Many people with cancer feel that they have lost control of their lives. The key point that we want you to take away from this chapter, is that there are things that you can do that will help you gain control of your life and manage stress.

Now let's look at some of the ways to gain control of your life and manage stress

It is important not to be lulled into a false sense of security by the 'homeostasis melancholy' discussed earlier. You now need to be smart at recognising that all issues need to be addressed. As you gradually address all the issues to do with your health a 'feeling of plenty of energy' becomes your new normal and you start to use homeostasis for your gradual health improvement.

Some specific actions that you can take to gain control of your life and manage stress are set out below:

Strategy 1 – Analyse your own behaviour

By analysing your own behaviour you may discover that you have built in 'Coping Mechanisms' that are actually designed to stop you changing. Sometimes it is also necessary to look at the coping mechanisms that others around you are using as much of your behaviour may be in response to those around you. Coping mechanisms are patterns of behaviour that we develop which help us deal with the world around us and allow us the feeling of comfort and normality (i.e. a mental form of homeostasis). When you visit your neighbourhood supermarket you tend to deal with the situation in a fixed pattern – you go down the same isles and pick up from the same shelves the same products that you buy every week. So you have developed a coping mechanism for dealing with the supermarket. To implement a healthy eating program you will definitely have to address this coping mechanism and work out a new way of coping with the weekly shopping. Other negative patterns of behaviour can develop that worsen our health condition, while positive coping mechanisms will enable us to easily manage the changes needed to steadily improve our health.

Some examples of negative coping mechanisms are:

- Drama patterns – 'the car has just been repossessed', 'the dog died', 'someone cut me off on the road' - whenever life threatens to go smoothly a little voice inside says 'this can't be right' and to prove it another drama quickly arises.
- Sickness patterns – as soon as good health is achieved another illness arises to prove that 'you are always sick'.
- Indispensable patterns – as soon as you train someone they leave, you are the only one that can do a job properly, people are lazy they never do their job properly – these all arise to prove that you are 'indispensable' when in fact the world will keep going quite happily whether you are around or not – to reinforce this negative pattern of behaviour people will often invent false standards of what is a good job just to prove that they are the only person who can do the job.
- Mess patterns – constantly living in a mess so that you can never find what you want or, alternatively, you are the only person who can find what you want – is a way of coping with the reality but always leads to failure.
- Cleanliness patterns - constantly cleaning can be a coping mechanism that blocks out other thoughts just as constantly being messy has the same result – a person who constantly cleans never achieves much else than a temporarily clean environment. Living in a clean environment is actually good and healthy but obsessing about it to the point where you don't have enough time to implement key health improvement actions creates a problem.

So gaining control of your life may often require us to learn new patterns of behaviour that become our new coping mechanisms. Whenever we decide to change we will always be challenged and meet resistance. Remember that the old pattern of behaviour has taken a long time to build up and is now effectively managed by your subconscious - change will not be easy. The week you decide to adopt a healthy eating program you can bet you will receive a number of invitations to dinners, cocktail parties, birthday parties, etc - just to see if you are serious about making the change.

So to make sure that the change is effective you may need to use some more of the other techniques and strategies we have listed below.

Strategy 2 – Develop a plan

Having a simple plan of what you want to achieve in your life gives you incredible drive. The feeling of having a purpose in life gives you a positive mind set which helps offset any negatives that may be around you. The nightly news that we see or hear is often so full of negatives that you could easily believe that the world is a terrible place full of bad people. Once you develop a plan for yourself it becomes a lot easier to put things in perspective and see that the negative news items are actually only about a very small portion of the world's population. If you get the opportunity to travel around the world you will start to realise that most people and places are not actually that bad and most people are actually working together to make the world a better place. When you develop a plan for your life and set some objectives you will quickly see that you can fit into this positive world of people working together to build a better world.

Strategy 3 – Implement Time Management Techniques

Common reasons given for not implementing a health improvement program are 'very tired', 'not enough time', and 'lack of self-discipline'. Healthy eating will put you into fat burning mode and creates lots of energy so the 'very tired' reason disappears. Time management techniques can be used to address 'not enough time' and 'lack of self-discipline'. So here are some actions that you may find useful:

- Focus – the most important reality of life is that 'What you focus on is what you get' – so if you focus on health improvement you will achieve good health, have lots of energy and look and feel healthy – you have to decide that this is your major focus.

- Use a 'To Do List'. Pick the hardest job on the list or the one you dislike doing and do it first. Getting this job out of the way will reduce stress for the rest of the day and make doing the other things feel easy. If you find exercise the hardest thing to implement you might decide to do this first thing every morning so that you feel good for the rest of the day that you are making progress.

- Break a major job down into simple tasks - doing each small simple task is a lot less stressful and easier to manage than working on one major job and never getting it finished – you will now see yourself steadily moving towards your objective one step at a time – so if you are allocated a major job at work which is very important to your career and you definitely want to do it and this may reduce your time available for health improvement then you need to break the new major job down into smaller parts and address the key issues first so that you can demonstrate you are making progress – this will give you plenty of time to fit in the health improvement tasks into your daily routine.

- Train and delegate – Many people think that they have to do every chore in the house or every key job in the work environment simply because they have experienced a situation in the past where someone has failed to do something properly. If you think like this you will never have time for a health improvement program. You need to develop skills in training and delegating so that you will have time for the most important task in your life – improving your health. When you train a person to do part of your work, make sure that you are confident that they really understand what to do and the outcomes expected and then leave them to it. You may need to occasionally check their output and do some retraining but your life will become a lot less stressful the more you do this. This works equally at home as well as at work - train the kids to make their beds and clean their rooms - check on them occasionally and praise their good work and retrain them if the results are not good.

- Keep life simple - always eliminate unnecessary complications - the simple ways of doing something are always the most effective and create the least stress and make more time available for implementing health improvement.

- Take notes when important matters come up - you can then deal with these issues when you have time and your mind can be free for the more immediate issues. Notes keep your mind free to focus on the most important issue in front of you – your health.

- Always be prepared - planning and preparation can always increase the amount of time we have available for the important things in life. Plan the key things you need to do at home and at work - focus on these and not all the minor issues that may arise to distract you.

- Take time to choose your response - if you are faced with an irate person you can choose whether you want to remain calm or you want to blow off steam like them. Either response may be appropriate. The important issue is that you have made the choice in advance and afterwards you don't need to dwell on the issue. You can quickly move on and focus back on the key issue – getting healthy. Remember one of the most important realities of life – 'What you focus on is what you get' – focus on getting healthy and you will achieve your goal.

- Build your self-worth. As you implement your health improvement actions you will start to look healthier and may even receive a few positive comments. Simply say 'Thank You' to positive complements as this builds your self-worth without sounding like you were just elected as President. Another technique is to praise in public and criticise in private - praising a person in public for something that has been well done will add to their self-worth as well as your self-worth. Telling someone about a poor outcome in private will give you the opportunity to talk confidentially about the issues and will keep both of you positive about the outcomes and thus diminishing the level of stress or embarrassment involved. This applies equally at home as well as at work – tell children about poor outcomes in private – not in front of other children or their friends.

- Learn to say 'No'. Over-commitment will almost always create more stress for you and everyone around you and leave little time for important issues like getting healthy. Know your limitations and work within them. By saying 'No' to others when something cannot realistically be achieved is being honest and creating certainty. You can then work with the person wanting to delegate work to you to find another way of achieving the outcome without you losing the time needed for your important goals.

- Be alert to procrastination in yourself and in others. Look for the reason that you or someone else is procrastinating and find a way of overcoming the issue.

- Don't be overwhelmed by emails, facebook activities or paperwork - sort out what is important and get rid of the rest. Look at ways of minimising what comes to you on a daily basis – remember 'What you focus on is what you get' – you now have the tools to focus on being healthy so make this your major focus.

Strategy 4 - Learn to Listen

Listening to another person very carefully so that you really understand what they are talking about is the best compliment that you can give to another person and will make your life incredibly easy and stress free. If you really understand the people around you then you will not be stressed by their behaviour or do things unintentionally that create negative situations. You can also explain your situation in terms that the other person will appreciate. So by listening you become an effective communicator. Effective communication is one of the keys to success in life and will help you implement a health improvement program. This is particularly important when you live with a group of people and you are the only one of the group motivated to improve your health. The others may not be enthusiastic about the change and may actually sabotage your efforts. So it is very important to fully understand the people around you so that you can implement health improvement in ways that creates the least difficulties for them. When others see the positive results in you they will then be enthusiastic to make the changes as well if you communicate in a way that they can relate to and feel positive about.

Strategy 5 - Think Win/Win

Life doesn't have to be full of situations where one person gets what they want at the expense of another person. By always thinking win/win you will be looking for ways that you can achieve what you want to and allow other people also to achieve what they want to at the same time. This may require a bit of thought but once you get into the habit of thinking like this it is amazing how quickly effective solutions arise. When you combine the 'Win/Win' thought pattern with the effective communication you get by 'Learning to Listen' you may find that many people around you also want to participate in health improvement. You may find that all the people around you become an effective support group as you and they go through the process of health improvement.

Strategy 6– Stress Reduction

The way your body responds to stress over time can be one of the underlying causes of why your body systems are out of balance. All the above strategies will help reduce the amount of stress in your life. The following are a few other ideas that may also help reduce stress:

- Get plenty of exercise – exercise reduces the effects of stress on your body.
- Have more fun – doing things that you enjoy will help you to relax.
- Express your feelings – unexpressed emotions are the building blocks of stress, pain, and illness.
- Get good sleep – poor sleep or sleep habits do not let your body really rest, discharge tensions and recharge.
- Learn relaxation exercises – these can help reduce stress through letting go of mental stresses and experiencing moments of inner peace.
- Develop good relationships – those who love and accept you, and will advise but not judge you, are your true friends.

Strategy 7 - Visualisations & Affirmations

We have talked about making health improvement the key objective in your life. Sometimes you have to convince your subconscious that you really do want to achieve this goal. We have developed the following technique that you can use to convince your subconscious that health improvement is your new goal. After achieving the great health and energy that you are after you may want to use this technique to achieve other things in your life.

Visualisation is a matter of picturing something in your mind. Affirmations are basically words that you repeat to yourself that focus your attention on a particular topic or outcome (they must be clear and precise to be effective). Meditation is a technique of stilling the mind.

For our clients we have combined visualisation, affirmation and meditation into one powerful technique. We call it – Perpetual Mind Rejuvenation. In addition to our cancer clients we also use this technique for our clients working on weight loss or following our anti-aging program called "Perpetual Rejuvenation" (visit us at www.perpetualrejuvenation.com for more information about our anti-aging program).

The following is an example of how it works – as you become experienced in the technique you can use it to achieve many positive outcomes in your life.

Find a quiet spot, sit still and use your mind as follows:

First count the number one to yourself slowly until all thoughts have gone and you are focusing only on the number one.

Next imagine red energy is coming from the earth below your feet and rising up into your legs and that this energy is giving you the stamina you need for today.

Feel the red energy convert to orange energy and allow it to rise up through your body and balance all the hormones in your body so you feel stable and energetic.

Now allow yellow energy from the sun to enter your body through your abdomen and feel it nourish your digestive system including your liver and pancreas.

Next breathe in the green energy of the trees and allow the oxygen to travel to every part of your body.

Imagine the gentle pounding of the ocean and add this blue energy to the blue energy of the sky and allow this blue energy to enter through your throat and let it travel down your spine relaxing each nerve in your body. When the blue energy reaches your toes allow it to travel back up your spine to your face and allow your face to relax and glow with vitality.

Next allow purple energy from the universe to enter through the top of your head so that you now feel totally connected with the whole universe and the knowledge of the universe is freely available to you.

Now allow your whole body to glow with a violet energy that allows you to fully connect with every aspect of the universe.

Finally, while you are fully connected to the universe allow whatever it is you desire to flow into your body – such as weight loss, perfect health, the cure of a disease, meeting the right person, wealth, happiness, development of a specific aspect of your business, removal of a bad habit, adoption of a good habit, etc, etc – but remember that you are using a powerful tool so select what you want carefully and only focus on one thing at a time (one thing in one session).

You can select the words for this final step in the form of an affirmation such as 'I am bringing my body into balance', 'My healing has already begun', 'I have more energy every day', 'My muscles are growing stronger as my fat reduces', 'I am willing to change', 'I love life', 'I love my body'.

Before you begin a Perpetual Mind Rejuvenation exercise think carefully about what it is that you most need to change in your life or what is most needed to add to your life to improve it. The objective can be simple or complex and the benefit does not necessarily have to be for you – your objective could be to improve your skill at helping others. When you establish your objective then carefully develop a phrase that explains it – this phrase should be absolutely clear to anybody who hears it so that it is absolutely clear what you want to happen.

You may want to use our technique of "Perpetual Mind Rejuvenation" to identify the aspect of your behaviour that they want to change and then define a new clear way of coping and use this as your affirmation. An example of an affirmation to change is "I will replace my drama coping mechanism with a 'to do' list which is always up to date with priorities allocated and I am successfully completing the next most important job – life is never a drama for me"

Money is an incredibly important issue for most people in the Western world. So let's have a look at how you would use the technique to improve your financial situation. A phrase like "I want more money" is not clear as this could mean one cent more, one dollar more, etc. However, a phrase like "My income will increase to $150,000 per annum by June next year" is absolutely clear. Be careful, though, that this is an achievable goal and that you have the health, energy and skills to achieve it. If your starting point is no job at all then you will need to start with an objective of getting a job. If you need more energy you might start with 'My energy levels will improve so that I can work 8 hours a day without getting tired or slowing down' or 'My skill levels will improve so that I am worth $100,000 a year in income' and then at a later stage when you have achieved the $100,000 a year level move up to $150,000.

Remember the whole Perpetual Mind Rejuvenation exercise should only focus on one thing at a time and it should be absolutely clear what you are trying to achieve. Also remember that good health is the basis for achieving all other objectives and your initial focus with Perpetual Mind Rejuvenation exercises should be on health improvement.

5 EATING HEALTHY

The food we eat can have a direct impact on getting cancer, preventing cancer, and the process for removing cancer from your body.

We are continually surprised about how many of our new clients do not appreciate the full impacts that foods have on our health.

Hippocrates (Greek physician c. 460 BC – 370 BC) earned the title of 'Father of Medicine' by creating moral and professional standards for physicians. He is also accredited with the quote – 'Let food be thy medicine and medicine be thy food'. Since then scientists have been uncovering thousands of links between food and health. While obesity is an obvious link, there are many less obvious. Food affects our mood, can trigger depression, is related to allergies, many cancers have been directly related to foods. Foods can trigger diarrhoea or constipation, can improve or reduce athletic performance, can trigger the release of hormones, can affect cardiovascular health, can affect our sleep, can impact on our ability to fight cold and flu and many other diseases, can give us food poisoning or help us overcome it, etc, etc. Most important is that food makes us feel good.

Healthy eating needs to become a habit for anyone wanting to achieve good health. As you gradually move away from foods high in sugar and high in saturated fats you find that your taste buds change and these foods eventually lose their addictive control over your eating. You become in control of your eating and you continually make healthy choices – in addition to being in control you also feel great.

Protein is the key to long term good health. Animal sources of protein are suitable for most people (including eggs, fish and meats) and where they are the main source of your protein they should be at least one third of what you eat. We find it easy to manage if you try to achieve this one third balance at every meal. All types of beans (legumes) are another good source of protein and can be used as alternatives at most meals. For vegetarians your major focus will be to obtain enough protein – you will need to be constantly alert as to whether the vegetable and grain sources that you are using are providing adequate amounts of protein.

Vegetables are essential. Virtually all the diets that we recommend are very high in vegetables because the scientific data keeps rolling in showing that they have incredible health benefits, especially when you eat a good variety every day. While the current Government recommendations in most countries are five serves of vegetables per day we recommend that you go well beyond this and try for six or seven servings per day.

A review carried out in 2007 of scientific studies[1] that looked at the association between vegetables and cancer risk showed that 80% of all studies had concluded that vegetables reduced the risk of cancer and in regard to raw vegetables it was 87%. From a science point of view this is overwhelming evidence as it is very rare to get such a high level of consistency in scientific studies.

A study[2] published in April 2010 looked at the health benefits of cruciferous vegetables and found that they were not just protective against cancer but also protective against cardiovascular disease. Another study[3] showed that blood pressure was better maintained by people eating vegetables regularly.

One of the great components of vegetables is their indigestible fibre. As fibre passes through the digestive system, it soaks up water like a sponge and expands. This can calm the irritable bowel and, by triggering regular bowel movements, can relieve or prevent constipation[4] as well as triggering a number of beneficial biochemical actions in the gastrointestinal system.

Eye health is another area that has been subject to investigation demonstrating a preventative effect of vegetables against macular degeneration and other eye health issues. Consumption of vegetables containing two carotenoid pigments may be linked to a reduced risk for age-related macular degeneration[5], the leading cause of vision loss in people over the age of 55. According to research[6], lutein and zeaxanthin comprise a component of the central region of the retina and may play a role in some aspects of visual acuity. Increasing the concentration of these pigments in the eye may prevent the devastating vision loss caused by age-related macular degeneration.

It would take a whole book to list all the benefits and all the research on vegetables – take it from us – a good variety of vegetables every day is an essential component of any health maintenance protocol.

Selecting vegetables by colour is a simple way of making sure you get a good variety of nutrients. Try to have at least one serving from every colour every day. One way of dividing vegetables into colours is set out below:

- Green – includes spinach, broccoli, lettuce, asparagus, peas, green beans, cabbage, Brussels sprouts, green olives.
- Orange/yellow – includes carrots, pumpkin, corn, and sweet potato.
- White/Brown – includes cauliflower, garlic, ginger, mushrooms, onions, chickpeas, and potatoes (note – only use potatoes if you need to gain weight or do more than five hours of physical work per day – otherwise avoid).
- Red – red capsicum, radishes and tomatoes (note – limit tomatoes as they are actually a fruit and contain reasonably high amounts of fructose which could worsen your condition).
- Purple/blue – beetroot, purple asparagus, red cabbage, olives, red onions.
- Multi-coloured – avocado, zucchini, egg plant, celery and beans can be a variety of colours.

By selecting a good variety of vegetables you are obtaining a good selection of carbohydrates, fats, fibre, protein, water, vitamins, minerals and phytochemicals. The study of phytochemicals in vegetables is progressing rapidly, with scientists uncovering another health improvement aspect, or disease fighting aspect virtually every day.

Good fats – the third essential component of healthy eating

Good fats are those found in foods such as fish, nuts, seeds and cold-pressed vegetable oils. A handful of nuts and seeds (around ¼ cup) daily should be enough for most people. About 2 tablespoons of a good oil (like cold pressed extra virgin olive oil) mixed with your food will provide the rest of your daily needs for good fats.

Cooking methods – stir fries, omelettes, slow cooking, steaming vegetables, frying in butter, stews and baking are all OK - avoid burning foods, bar-b-q's, etc as this may stimulate carcinogenic activity – check with cookware suppliers that you are not using cookware that may leach metals into foods.

Slow Cooking – An easy way to good health

We constantly promote the benefits of whole foods cooked in a healthy way. Slow cooking is a great way to combine a good source of protein with lots of vegetables and your favourite herbs. Slow cooking can be done in the slow cooker, on the stove top or in the oven.

There is something wonderful and comforting about slow-cooked food. The sensational aroma fills your house with a sense of wellbeing and the irresistible rich flavours provide comfort to every part of your mind, body and spirit. Best of all slow-cooked food practically cooks itself – especially if you use a slow cooker. Just throw all the ingredients in the slow cooker in the morning, switch it on and come home in the evening to a welcoming aroma at the door and dinner ready.

There are thousands of slow-cooker recipes available on the internet – just pick one that contains healthy ingredients or modify it to suit your needs.

'Carbs' for Exercise

Thus healthy eating consists mainly of good protein sources plus vegetables plus a small amount of good fats. For most people this will supply adequate amounts of carbohydrates for all your energy needs. So most people can live without grains, sugar, dairy products, fruit, junk food, cookies, cakes, sweets, sweetened drinks, etc, etc. However, if you plan on doing more than one hour of aerobic exercise per day then you will need some additional sources of carbohydrates to burn up – a simple way to gauge this is to add one piece of fruit for every 45 minutes of additional exercise that you plan to do and see if this keeps your energy levels up and weight in balance. Fruit is best consumed between meals as the metabolism of the fructose in the fruit may interfere with the normal processes of metabolising other foods (see our book 'FEAR Made You Fat & Not Calories' for more details on this topic).

Water is the fourth key ingredient that you need to support healthy eating.

You need water for the repair processes and for the health of all body systems. Most people will need between one to two litres of water per day. You need to be at the higher end of scale on hot days and if exercising more than normal and the more exercise the more water that you will need. It is best to drink away from meals.

Cereals, grains & dairy

We have left cereals, grains and dairy to later in the discussion because a) you can achieve a balanced diet without them and b) they create the most allergies so they are not for everyone. The effects of an allergy on your health should not be underestimated. An allergy can easily block the absorption of key nutrients and be the underlying reason for the start of your poor health, including the eventual development of cancer.

For the average person living in a developed country and doing less than one hour of aerobic exercise per day, the eating of grains is unnecessary and will be stored as fat instead of being burned off as per its function. Any farmer knows that if you want to fatten up cattle then your feed them grains – it is exactly the same with people who don't exercise.

If you are doing enough exercise to eat grains or need to include them because you are a vegetarian, then look for "ancient" grains such as spelt, kumat, oats, rye, and barley. Spelt, rye and other ancient grain breads are available at some supermarkets and bakeries. To find a healthy commercially available breakfast cereal you will need to do some research to find out what is available in your area – most commercially available breakfast cereals have modified grains and are loaded with sugar and are definitely on the 'Avoid' list when you have cancer.

Dairy

For most people 'milk' means cow's milk but there are a number of issues to consider.

A big issue is pasteurization. Pasteurization is usually carried out using continuous-flow equipment, which gives a treatment of at least 72°C for 15 seconds, which is sufficient to kill all non-sporing pathogens and non-thermoduric organisms. The resistance of spores is one reason why milk needs to be stored at refrigeration temperatures to prevent the growth of sporing organisms. Pasteurization was introduced at a time when farming practices produced unhealthy milk and gave the dairy industry an excuse for not cleaning up their act. With current knowledge farmers could produce healthy milk without the need for pasteurization. Various enzymes are deactivated with heat including - gamma-glutamyltransferase, alkaline phosphatase and lactate dehydrogenase. The degree of deactivation of alkaline phosphatase is actually used as a test of how effective the pasteurization has been. A study[7] published in November 2010 found that intestinal alkaline phosphatase preserves the normal homeostasis of gut microbiota and recommends consideration for supplementation with alkaline phosphatase especially after use of antibiotics. Seems a little strange that scientists are now recommending we put back in our diet something that food scientists have been taking out of our diet for years. Having a balanced gut bacteria is one of the key issues in maintaining a balanced immune system, preventing cancer and preventing allergies although, of course, many other issues are involved. There only seems to be two ways to go with pasteurization – 1) after pasteurization put back into the milk all the good things that have been destroyed or 2) get the farmers to produce milk that we can drink so we don't need pasteurization. The 'do nothing' option will not be good for maintaining health and means we need to look to other alternatives to cow's milk. So for most people with cancer, cow's milk is on the 'Avoid' list.

Another big issue with milk (as with most dairy products) is that it contains lactose. Lactose intolerance is probably the most common food intolerance throughout the world. To tolerate lactose you need to produce an enzyme in your small intestine called, lactase. Lactase is present predominantly along the brush border membrane of the differentiated enterocytes, lining the villi of the small intestine, and is encoded by the LCT gene. Deficiency in lactase can arise genetically, but more commonly arises as we age. It seems that genetically we were intended to only drink milk when we were young. However, some people have an altered genetic structure which allows them to tolerate milk all their life. The symptoms of lactose intolerance include cramps, bloating, wind and diarrhoea. If you have these symptoms after drinking milk then get checked out for lactose intolerance.

Lactose intolerance should not be confused with milk allergy which is related to milk proteins. The reaction to cow's milk proteins can be immediate or delayed up to 48 hours. It is associated with vomiting, chronic diarrhoea, eczema, and failure to thrive. The allergy section in this book explains tests that you can do to be assessed for food allergies and intolerances like milk protein allergy.

Some people who cannot tolerate cow's milk, can tolerate goat's milk and so it is regarded as a 'gentler' alternative.

The proteins in either goat's milk, or cow's milk, can be useful in some diets for people who do not have cancer. Milk is also a valuable source of saturated fats for those not getting them from any other source. Low fat milks and all the other varieties of altered milks are not recommended because of the processes used to alter milk.

Yogurts (fermented milk) usually contain all the constituents present in the original milk, with the exception of the lactose which is substantially reduced. For people who can tolerate milk products, yogurt can be a valuable addition to the diet. However, you need to be careful with product selection as many brands have artificially added sugars, flavourings, etc. You need to look for a natural yoghurt with nothing added.

Dietary Fibre – Are you getting the active ingredients?

A number of very unpleasant conditions have been associated with diets lacking in dietary fibre, including many diseases of the gastrointestinal system, constipation, gall bladder disease, coronary artery disease, diabetes, obesity and some cancers. The active ingredients in dietary fibre include cellulose, gums, hemicelluloses, lignin, mucilage, pectin substances, plant sterols and saponins. For our clients we focus on vegetables and some fruits as the primary sources of dietary fibre but where the client needs and can tolerate grains then we will also include whole grain cereals. The biggest issue with cereals is that, the vast majority of those available in the supermarket have significantly depleted active ingredients as a result of food processing and refining. It is essential to seek out products that have not been modified and retain the active ingredients.

Folic Acid – An essential nutrient

Folic acid is one of those essential nutrients that is often depleted by our modern lifestyle.

The main sources of folic acid are beans, eggs, green leafy vegetables and lentils.

The demand in the body for folic acid can be increased as you age, by consumption of alcohol, inadequate protein intake (particularly if it results in vitamin B12 deficiency), diarrhoea, some forms of anaemia, some cancers and other chronic diseases, and also pregnancy and lactation deplete reserves of folic acid. Inadequate amounts of folic acid can result in premature and low birth weight infants and retardation.

Some of the important body functions facilitated by folic acid are nucleic acid synthesis and metabolism, DNA repair, growth, maturation of blood cells and the synthesis of noradrenaline, serotonin and choline. Thus a variety of functions throughout our body are affected in some way by folic acid, including our ability to resist chronic disease and cancer as we age, our ability to respond to stress and even our ability to feel happy (serotonin).

Some healthy eating tips

- A stir fry is a simple way of getting a good variety of vegetables in one meal.
- Garlic, ginger, mushrooms, onions, spinach, etc can be added to lots of meals including omelettes and frittatas.
- Increase the variety in salads by adding to the traditional salad vegetables others such as- baby spinach, rocket, lightly steamed broccoli, red capsicum, roast sweet potato, butterbeans or chickpeas.
- Take a salad to work for lunch, instead of buying a take away.
- Grate or dice onion, carrot, zucchini, red capsicum and corn into a savoury muffin mixture.
- Have vegetable sticks such as carrot and celery on hand for a healthy snack, and these can be eaten with hummus.
- For optimal health and wellness it is always best to eat seasonal, fresh, biodynamic or organic foods. Foods that are processed have very little nutritional value, have lost all their vitality and may detract from your wellness.

- Keep carbohydrates found in bread, rice, pasta, and potato to a minimum and when they are included make sure they are whole grains and not refined foods.
- Always take time to sit down and enjoy your meal. Chew each mouthful well, as digestion begins in the mouth, and savour the wonderful, healthy food that you are providing for your body.
- Eat regularly, at least every four to five hours, as our body needs regular fuel to function at optimal levels. Skipping meals may result in low blood sugar, slow metabolism, fatigue, poor concentration and feeling unwell.
- Try not to drink too much fluid with your meal as this may slow digestion – water and herbal teas are best taken between meals.
- Stop eating when you begin to feel full to give your body time to assimilate the food and acknowledge that you have eaten enough.
- Participate in the meal planning process and try and prepare as many of your meals as possible. When you take the time to fully participate in the meal preparation you are nourishing not only your body but also your soul. The more you do this the more you will gain from the culinary experience. It really is a delight!
- Aim to eat at least one raw food group every day, unless your practitioner advises otherwise. Many raw foods, especially vegetables and fruits, contain enzymes and nutrients that are destroyed in the cooking process, hence eating them raw will add to your vitality and stamina.
- Participate in regular exercise between meals. A walk around the park, running in the back yard with the children, doing a few skips on the rope. Whatever it is, get active! Regular physical movement assists all aspects of our health, from body strength, organ function and waste elimination to mental and spiritual wellbeing and so helps make sure you get the best benefits from the food you have eaten.

References

1. Beliveau R, et al, 2007, Role of nutrition in preventing cancer, *Canadian Family Physician*, 53: 1905-1911, PMID: 18000267
2. Shan Y, et al, 2010, Protective Effect of Sulforaphane on Human Vascular Endothelial Cells Against Lipopolysaccharide-Induced Inflammatory Damage, *Cardiovascular Toxicology*, PMID: 20405237

3. Appel LJ, et al, 1997, A clinical trial of the effects of dietary patterns on blood pressure, DASH Collaborative Research Group, *New England Journal Medicine*, 336:1117–24, PMID: 9099655

4. Lembo A, Camilleri M, 2003, Chronic constipation, *New England Journal Medicine*, 349:1360–68, PMID: 14523145

5. Bernstein PS, 2009, Nutritional Interventions against Age-Related Macular Degeneration, *Acta Hortic*, 841:103-112, PMID: 20190863

6. Ma L, Lin XM, 2010, Effects of lutein and zeaxanthin on aspects of eye health, *J Sci Food Agric*, 90(1):2-12, PMID: 20355006

7. Malo MS, et al, 2010, Intestinal alkaline phosphatase preserves the normal homeostasis of gut microbiota, *Gut*, 59(11), 1476-84, PMID: 20947883

6 FOODS TO AVOID WHEN YOU HAVE CANCER

In the previous chapter we outlined the key ingredients for a healthy eating plan and mentioned that some foods should be avoided when you have cancer.

The following is the list of foods to avoid:

- All red meats – we are trying to limit the availability of iron to the cancer. However, there may be some circumstances where your nutritional advisor will say that red meat is OK.
- All cereals and grain especially breads, cakes, biscuits, crackers, donuts, chips, bagels, pizza, rice dishes, spaghetti, rice puddings, lasagne, linguine, muffins, macaroni, and pastries – all these feed cancers. If you are a vegetarian you will need to include grains to get the full range of proteins, so use 'ancient grains' as set out in the previous chapter.
- Sugary items – including soft drinks, fruit juices, honey, jam, sugar, lollies, chocolate, sherbet, milkshakes, fruitcakes, marshmallow, pancake syrup, muesli, and jelly – all these feed cancers. However, a small amount of dark chocolate is OK to include as a treat.
- Potatoes - including sweet potatoes, white potatoes, yams and potato salads – all these feed cancers.
- Fruits including apples, oranges, peaches, cantaloupe (rockmelon), kiwi fruit, fruit juices, bananas, mangoes, pears, plums, prunes, raisins, dates, pineapple, nectarines, grapes, melons and berries – all these feed cancers. You may include some mixed berries for their antioxidant effect but only between meals.

- Dairy Products – as set out in the previous chapter, the majority of people with cancer need to avoid dairy products.
- Avoid all alcohol because you need your liver to work at maximum capacity so that any parts of the cancer that your body sends to the liver can be processed and removed from your body and as we have demonstrated elsewhere in this book. Also alcohol can reduce the amount of protein that is transported in your blood.
- Avoid all smoked/cured foods (note – sodium nitrate is converted to nitrosamine, a carcinogen added to processed meats, so avoid ham, bacon, pickled, fried or smoked foods).
- Avoid bar-b-q or any form of cooking that burns food.
- Avoid all deep fried foods including chips, spring rolls and doughnuts.
- Any foods containing Artificial Trans Fats - After about 20 years of inaction, governments around the world have started to take specific actions about artificial trans fats and most countries now have some controls over artificial trans fats. Unfortunately, some countries like the United States haven't required the removal of trans fats from all foods but require the food to be labelled if the trans fat content is more than 0.5 grams. This means in the US the label can read zero trans fats if the quantity is less than 0.5 grams which means that you could be unknowingly consuming 0.49 grams of trans fats in four different products and thus consume 1.96 grams of trans fats in a single day. The US Food and Drug Administration recommends that healthy individuals do not exceed a daily maximum of 1.11 grams. However, for people with cancer you cannot afford to risk any exposure to artificial trans fats and they should be avoided altogether.
- Excessive amounts of saturated fats – small amounts of saturated fats that appear naturally in foods like meats are OK but excessive amounts added to foods will place an unnecessary burden on your body while you are trying to get healthy – so avoid excessive amounts of saturated fats.
- Based on the above, the majority of processed foods need to be avoided.
- Coffee – keep in moderation – maximum of 2 cups per day

Concerns about a low carbohydrate diet

A frequently cited concern with avoiding all the above foods is that a low carbohydrate diet has the potential for increased renal disease because of the resulting high protein content of the diet. If the diet is balanced properly with vegetables this is never an issue. A study[1] published in April 2010 shows that a very low carbohydrate diet (much lower than the ones we use) does not adversely affect renal function.

The Restricted Ketogenic Diet

By combining our healthy eating guidelines (the foods to eat) in the previous chapter with the 'food to avoid' list you come close to what some researchers call the 'Restricted Ketogenic Diet'. Recent research has shown that this diet can restrict the sources of glucose and glutamine that feed cancers and thus be an effective part of managing the disease[2]. Other recent research has shown that a ketogenic diet is suitable for patients with advanced cancer[3]. This diet may also work well in conjunction with some drugs like metformin[4] to completely restrict the source of nutrients that feed cancers so it could be worth discussing this strategy with your doctor.

Weaning Yourself Off the Sweet Taste

As you can see from the above list the biggest issue for people with cancer is to wean themselves off the sweet taste. A research paper[3] published in 2007 confirmed what we all know – sugar is incredibly addictive and actually more addictive than cocaine.

Refined sugars such as sucrose and fructose were absent in the diet of most people until recently in human history (beginning with the post World War Two food processing revolution/disaster). The researchers note that overconsumption of diets rich in sugars contributes together with other factors to drive the increase in chronic disease. Overconsumption of sugar-dense foods or beverages is initially motivated by the pleasure of sweet taste, and can be directly compared with drug addiction. The research was carried out on rats but can be related to humans and showed that 94% of animals including even cocaine addicted animals preferred the sweet taste to a dose of cocaine. The research showed that a dependence-like state appeared to be induced by sugar-dense foods and beverages.

Here are some tips on how to wean yourself off the sweet taste:

- Start with a substitute - Use Herbs & Spices instead of Sugar – when cooking it may be possible to use herbs and spices instead of sugar even if the recipe calls for sugar – when buying processed food look for foods that have used herbs and spices and contain no or little sugar.

- Use cooking techniques that don't take much time but bring out the real flavours of food like stir fries and slow cooking.
- Start appreciating the genuine flavours in whole foods and particularly vegetables – once you start to enjoy eating vegetables your desire for the sweet taste will diminish.
- Shop Where Whole Foods are Sold – shopping at the butcher, fishmonger and fruit and vegetable barn will provide you with all the healthy ingredients you need for a week of meals and so you don't even need to pass the tempting displays of sweetened food.
- Read labels or check on the internet before you buy any processed food or drink.
- Devote time to enjoying the pleasures of eating the food in front of you and don't allow distractions to spoil this great enjoyment in life.
- Give your palate time to change. You'll gradually lose your taste for excessively sweet foods – so give yourself time to adjust – the end result is fantastic.
- If you live in a country that has traditional healthy foods, then enjoy the experience of following the traditions of your ancestors. Don't be fooled by the advertising or packaging of products as this does not make the product healthy. If some of the traditions need a slight modification to make them more healthy then make the change. The recipes for traditional healthy food have been modified steadily over time as knowledge improves. This is not breaking tradition but being part of the tradition of preparing healthy food.

References

1. Brinkworth GD, et al, 2010 Apr, Renal function following long-term weight loss in individuals with abdominal obesity on a very-low-carbohydrate diet vs. high-carbohydrate diet, *Journal American Diet Association*, 110(4):633-8, PMID: 20338292
2. Sayfried TN, et al, 2011, Is the restricted ketogenic diet a viable alternative to the standard of care for managing malignant brain cancer? *Epilepsy Res*, 2011 Aug 30. [Epub ahead of print], PMID: 21885251

3. Schmidt M, et al, 2011, Effects of a ketogenic diet on the quality of life in 16 patients with advanced cancer: A pilot trial, *Nutr Metab (Lond)*, 8(1):54, PMID: 21794124
4. Oleksvszym J, 2011, The complete control of glucose level utilizing the composition of ketogenic diet with the gluconeogenesis inhibitor, the anti-diabetic drug metformin, as a potential anti-cancer therapy, *Med Hypotheses*, 77(2):171-3, PMID: 21530093
5. Lenoir M, et al, 2007, Intense Sweetness Surpasses Cocaine Reward, *PLoS ONE*, 2(8): e698, doi:10.1371/journal.pone.0000698

7 MANAGING YOUR ENVIRONMENT & REDUCE YOUR TOXIC LOAD

The environment in which you live is a critical element in how you manage your health. The food we eat is critical, but many other aspects of the environment need to be considered. A simple thing like living in an uncluttered house can make you feel positive and energetic. Some of the more complex issues are set out in this chapter.

Are toxins preventing you from obtaining good health?

There is a growing body of research indicating that the amount of toxins that our body has to deal with is increasing steadily. One study[1] in the United States ranked polycyclic aromatic hydrocarbon, benzene, acetaldehyde, and 1,3-butadiene as posing the greatest risk for cancer coming from outdoor air sources, whereas indoor air sources of cancer risk were primarily from chloroform, formaldehyde, and naphthalene risks.

The key to good health in this polluted environment is to have our body systems capable of dealing with the toxins, and disposing of them effectively. One of the organs that is key in this process is the liver. Liver detoxification of toxins happens in two phases. Phase 1 comprises mainly the cytochrome P450 super family of enzymes that binds with the foreign compound. Phase 2 involves the conversion of these compounds into water soluble compounds that can be excreted through the urine or bile. If the toxin arrives in the gastrointestinal system, healthy intestinal cells are also able to trigger phase 1 detoxification. Having a healthy gut flora is also essential to maintaining and supporting the detoxification process.

At our clinic we support the detoxification process by using nutrients that support the rejuvenation of the gastrointestinal cells, the liver cells and also support maintenance of a balanced gut flora. In our modern polluted environment this support process needs to be ongoing.

Research[2] published in January 2010 links Perfluorooctanoic acid (PFOA) and perfluoroctane sulphonate (PFOS) with people who have current thyroid disease. PFOA and PFOS are compounds with many industrial and consumer uses including most non-stick cookware and stain- and water-resistant coatings for carpets and fabrics. So if you already have thyroid disease then it is important that you avoid items containing PFOA and PFOS.

For the rest of us, this is another reason why we need to maintain our health in pristine condition. With our gastrointestinal system, liver and kidneys in top working order we have a good chance of detoxifying and removing from our bodies all the environmental toxins as they arrive.

Are food additives preventing you from obtaining good health?

The Australian Government like other governments around the world sets standards for food additives. These specify the safe level of an additive if consumed over a lifetime and restricts usage to that necessary to achieve the function of the additive. More information is available at www.foodstandards.gov.au

The issues that arise are that we are relying on a) tests performed on healthy individuals or on healthy cells in a laboratory, b) each additive is tested in isolation and not in combination with the 100's of other additives, and c) the background knowledge available to scientists changes rapidly over time but governments do not have the resources to constantly update the tests on additives based on new knowledge.

There is no question that less is best with artificial food additives. The best way for us to keep our consumption down is to avoid processed food as much as possible and consume instead fresh vegetables supported by adequate protein and fats.

Our body has natural mechanisms to dispose of unwanted food additives but these mechanisms only work properly if we are healthy.

It seems a contradiction but the reality is that you have to get healthy by not eating processed food so that you will be healthy enough to survive it when you do eat it.

Sugar may be bad, but some artificial sweeteners can be deadly

We recommend that all our clients avoid sweetened drinks of any kind – whether the sweetener be sugar, fructose or any other form of artificial sweetener. Although fructose can be a healthy ingredient when consumed as part of a whole fruit away from other food, the effect on our body changes dramatically when extracted from food and then artificially added in significant quantities to foods and drinks.

Research published in the Journal of Clinical Investigation[3] found that consuming drinks sweetened with fructose not only increased overall fat levels, it added to visceral fat (abdominal fat). The researchers also found that fructose specifically increases hepatic de novo lipogenesis, promotes dyslipidemia, and decreases insulin sensitivity, thus making individuals consuming these drinks more likely to be diabetic, obese and subject to the early onset of many chronic diseases including cancer.

If you think there are safe sweetened drinks try this exercise – note down the ingredients and particularly the identification number of each additive – then try googling each additive individually. Select some of the research that has been published in respected journals and peer reviewed.

It won't take long – you will reach the same conclusion as us – there are no sweetened drinks that support a healthy lifestyle – even the ones labelled 'health' drink.

The way you manage sleep could decide your level of health

Research published in 2001[4] provided conclusive evidence that chronic insomnia is directly associated with elevated blood levels of the stress hormones – ACTH and cortisol. It is known that chronic activation of the hypothalamic-pituitary-adrenal axis puts the chronic insomniac at high risk of anxiety, depression, reduced immunity, weight gain and many other chronic diseases. The researchers recommended that clinicians look for the underlying causes of the arousal of the hypothalamic-pituitary-adrenal axis as the basis for treatment.

The medical profession is so overwhelmed with patient numbers that they largely ignored this advice and stay with quick fix sleep promoting agents rather than treating the underlying cause. This is, of course, encouraged by the drug companies because it is not hard to figure out that you can make more money if you keep supplying people with sleeping pills rather than actually correct the underlying cause in a way that they don't need sleeping pills anymore. Just have a look at the drug company's own websites and you will be alarmed at the reported side effects and the potential for dependency on this type of drug. Of course, there may be occasions where short term use of a sleep promoting agent is justified, and has a desirable medical outcome, but the best medical outcome is always to look for the underlying cause.

So when looking for the underlying cause of the chronic activation of the hypothalamic-pituitary-adrenal axis you need to look at many aspects of health including the following issues:

- Diet – overconsumption of sugar and other inflammatory foods can put the body into a state of chronic inflammation and a chronic need for high insulin levels which combines to result in chronic elevation of the stress hormones.
- Drinks – overconsumption of stimulants like coffee and alcohol can have short term overstimulation of the stress hormones.
- Stressed Adrenal Glands – these can be stressed for a number of reasons and lead to elevated levels of stress hormones and for some people insomnia can actually be an early stage of chronic fatigue because the constant stimulation of the adrenal gland can eventually result in a decline in its functionality.
- Hormonal changes – especially those associated with menopause – can directly lead to a constant stimulation of the stress response and insomnia – moderating the hormonal changes by improving diet and health well before the onset of hormonal changes, is the way to minimise the effects of hormonal changes on sleep.
- Nutrient deficiencies – various nutrient deficiencies can result in overstimulation of stress hormones.
- Being overweight – is associated with dietary stimulation of stress hormones and sleep apnoea.

- Lack of exercise – regular exercise (but not immediately before sleep) can moderate the stress response and thus reduce levels of stress hormones.
- Environmental issues associated with sleep disturbance include – too much light in the room, a noisy partner, outside noise, electrical equipment in the bedroom, irregular sleeping hours, shift work, eating before bed, working before sleep, watching television immediately before sleep, low exposure to sunlight during the day can result in inadequate production of hormones needed for sleep, etc.

While the underlying causes can be many, and any person suffering from insomnia is likely to have more than one cause, it is not impossible to work through the issues, improving many aspects of health and resulting in good sleep being achieved – without the need for sleeping pills.

Prescription medications & over the counter drugs and vitamins

Our modern world is full of potential dangerous substances that can be found in most bathroom cupboards – including prescription medications and drugs, vitamins and minerals sold over the counter in supermarkets and pharmacies.

The main issues with these substances are side effects resulting from long term use (continuous use for more than three months) and the interactions that can arise when you take more than one substance per day. The authorities who test the safety of these substances do not usually monitor the effects of taking the substances over time and definitely do not test them in conjunction with the other cocktail of substances that are available over the counter. For most substances the supplier has a website with very useful information on the side effects if taken over longer periods – this information is freely available to anyone who wants to look – but unfortunately not many people including medical practitioners take the time to do this investigation.

Another issue to consider is the way that tablets are made. Other ingredients are added in addition to the main active ingredient. Binders, lubricants, coatings, disintegrants, and other excipients are the ingredients most commonly added by tablet manufacturers. These ingredients are added to make the tablet stay together, to make it shiny, and to make it break apart. Tablets are made in machines called tablet presses, which compact the powdered nutrients together (that have already been mixed with binders and lubricants) with a tremendous amount of force. Then, to make them shiny and easier to swallow, the tablets are often sprayed with shellac, like the shellac found on furniture, but it's labelled 'pharmaceutical glaze', or coated with a 'vegetable protein', most often a protein derived from corn.

So if you want long term good health you need to be careful about how you manage prescription medications, over the counter drugs and all the other vitamins, minerals, herbs and other substances found in supermarkets, health food shops and elsewhere.

Multi-vitamins & Breast Cancer

Many of you will have read the media reports in regard to a possible link between breast cancer and multi-vitamin use. The study[5] referred to by the media was the first study to draw any link between multi-vitamin use and breast cancer, whereas previous studies had demonstrated that there was no link.

The study published in the American Journal of Clinical Nutrition was data collected from 35,329 women enrolled in the Swedish Mammography Cohort study and was extracted via a mail out self-administered questionnaire in 1997, which covered multivitamin use as well as other known breast cancer risk factors. The women were followed up until 2007, with cases of invasive breast cancer recorded from relevant cancer registries in Sweden. The study is subject to many potential errors, including the relevance of recalling whether you had taken multi-vitamins and no detail recorded about actual quantities or types taken. Consequently no one should be concerned as a result of this study. However, it is a reminder about what we have been advising clients for a long time – do not self administer any over the counter product for any extended period of time.

We have adopted the common sense approach in regard to multi-vitamins and, in fact, all substances purchased over the counter – anyone who self administers any over the counter substance for any extended period of time is taking a risk with their health. Your body simply does not expect to receive high doses of any substance for an extended period of time. Of course, some people have special health needs and may need to supplement for a long period of time but it essential that this be under the supervision of a qualified practitioner.

Mobile phone - brain cancer risk

The evidence has been mounting over the last few years that there is an association between mobile phone use and brain cancer. Previous research has focused on periods under 3 years, but when you start to look at usage over 10 years the data starts to become alarming. Two research papers, by respected researchers in peer reviewed journals, have confirmed the link, and leave little doubt that prolonged mobile phone use increases your risk of developing brain cancer.

The first research paper[6] by researchers from the Australian National University, published their paper in the Journal of Surgical Neurology in September 2009, entitled 'Cell phones and brain tumours: a review including long-term epidemiologic data'. The researchers concluded that there is adequate epidemiologic evidence to suggest a link between prolonged cell phone usage and the development of an ipsilateral brain tumour. The data achieved statistical significance for glioma (a common form of brain tumour with increasing incidence) and acoustic neuroma (usually benign intracranial tumour).

The second research paper[7] by researchers from the Department of Oncology, Orebro University Hospital, Sweden, published their paper in the International Journal of Oncology in July 2009, entitled 'Mobile phones, cordless phones and the risk of brain tumours'. These researchers found that for astrocytoma and acoustic neuroma the highest risk was after 10 years of mobile phone use, and was the highest in people who had commenced use when they were under 20 years of age. This was followed up with further research[8] in 2010 which confirmed the previous findings.

Preventative action is needed now to prevent you becoming one of the statistics.

It is commonly known that many brain surgeons refuse to put a mobile phone to their head and only use the speaker phone – be careful, though, that you are not exposing the phone microwaves to another part of your body. Australian brain surgeons, Doctors Teo and Khurana, have expressed strong personal opinions in the media and publicly about mobile phones and brain cancer, and advocate precaution based on their concerns. This advice did not differ from the World Health Organisation's advice, which says, 'If individuals are concerned, they might choose to limit their own or their

41

children's RF exposure by limiting the length of calls, or by using hands-free devices to keep mobile phones away from the head and body' (WHO Fact Sheet No. 193).

The evidence about mobile phones is so strong that the World Health Organisation (WHO) has come to the same conclusion as the researchers. During May 2011 a group of scientists from 14 countries came to the International Agency for Research on Cancer (IARC) in France, to assess the potential carcinogenic hazards from exposure to radiofrequency electromagnetic fields associated with mobile phone use and from other devices. The resulting WHO announcement classified radiofrequency electromagnetic fields as possibly carcinogenic to humans.

Below are some of the simple things that you can do:

- Never let a child place a mobile phone anywhere near their head.
- Always use the speaker facility instead of putting the phone to your head.
- Keep all mobile phone calls to a minimum length of time and divert the mobile to a land line when you don't need it.
- Stay healthy so you can cope with radiation when you are exposed.

It is commonly known that being healthy reduces your risk of developing all forms of cancer. This is because malignancies start at a cellular level and healthy people have a defence mechanism that can identify malignant cells, and deal with them before they get out of control. However, constant repeat use that is triggering malignancies can easily overcome the body's natural defence mechanism.

Because we are exposed to many sources of radiation including mobile phones, it makes sense to improve your body's defence mechanisms that protect you against cancer formation and proliferation. If you are reading this book to develop a preventative program against cancer you may want to consider using Resveratrol as a supplement (possibly for one week per month rather than every day). Research[9] published in September 2009 in the Journal of Current Drug Metabolism, has provided further confirmation to the growing body of research, supporting Resveratrol as an extremely effective way of supporting our body's defence mechanisms against malignancies and other health issues.

Some more ideas for reducing your exposure to toxins

The toxic load on your body can be reduced but not eliminated by implementing some of the following ideas:

- Reduce the amount of scented products you have in your home or office – including perfumes, colognes, after-shaves, personal-care products, air fresheners, etc. Be careful about certain 'unscented' products that use 'masking fragrance' to cover up the original fragrance – these are doubly toxic.
- See if you can find unscented and environmentally friendly washing powders, fabric softeners, bleaches, detergents, etc.
- Be careful about the use of pesticides, fungicides, herbicides, and fertilizers. Pesticides can contain neuro-toxins (affect the central nervous system) – not something you want to spray on yourself or be breathing in while you are asleep.
- See if you can find non-toxic cleaning products and personal-care products.
- Consider installing water filters - either the reverse osmosis type or a water distillation system may be most effective.
- Eat organic food (food grown without pesticides or fertilizers) as often as possible.
- Wash all vegetable and fruits unless you are going to peel them, even organic produce.
- Avoiding processed foods will considerably cut down your toxic load.
- Check the clothing and other fabrics that you buy or have in your house to make sure they have not been treated with a toxic substance. Some 'permanent press' or 'wrinkle resistant' fabrics have been treated with formaldehyde. You want to keep your exposure to this toxic substance to an absolute minimum. It is likely to be in resins and other materials in your house or office[1] so don't add more exposure.
- Store food in glass containers as much as possible and avoid food and water stored in plastics, plastic wrap, polystyrene and other substances containing styrene. One study[10] found that styrene continuously leached from plastic water bottles making them less safe than unfiltered drinking water.

- Open your windows as often as possible. Even in the most polluted cities, the outdoor air has been found to be less toxic than the indoor air.

References

1. Loh MM, et al, 2007, Ranking cancer risks of organic hazardous air pollutants in the United States, *Environ Health Perspect*, 115(8):1160-8, PMID: 17687442
2. Melzer D, et al, 2010, Association Between Serum Perfluoroctanoic Acid (PFOA) and Thyroid Disease in the NHANES Study, *Environ Health Perspect*, [Epub ahead of print], PMID: 20089479
3. Stanhope KL, et al, 2009, Consuming fructose-sweetened, not glucose-sweetened, beverages increases visceral adiposity and lipids and decreases insulin sensitivity in overweight/obese humans, *Journal of Clinical Investigation*, 119(5), pp.1322-1334, PMCID: PMC2673878
4. Vgontzas AN, et al, 2001, Chronic insomnia is associated with nyctohemeral activation of the hypothalamic-pituitary-adrenal axis: clinical implications, *Journal of Clinical Endocrinological Metabolism*, 86(8):3787-94, PMID: 11502812
5. Larsson SC, et al, 2010, Multivitamin use and breast cancer incidence in a prospective cohort of Swedish women, *American Journal of Clinical Nutrition*, 91(5):1268-72, PMID: 20335555
6. Khurana VG, et al, 2009, Cell phones and brain tumors: a review including long-term epidemiologic data, *Journal of Surgical Neurology*, 72(3): 205-14, PMID: 19328536
7. Hardell L and Carlberg M, 2009, Mobile phones, cordless phones and the risk of brain tumours, *International Journal of Oncology*, 35(1): 5-17, PMID: 19513546
8. Hardell L, et al, 2010, Mobile phone use and the risk of malignant brain tumours: a case-control study on deceased cases and controls, *Neuroepidemiology*, 35(2): 109-14, PMID: 20551697
9. Brisdelli F, et al, 2009, Resveratrol: a Natural Polyphenol with Multiple Chemoproventative Properties, *Journal of Current Drug Metabolism*, 10(6): 530-46, PMID: 19702558
10. Ahmad M, Bajahlan AS, 2007, Leaching of styrene and other aromatic compounds in drinking water from PS bottles, *J Environ Sci (China)*, 19(4): 421-6, PMID: 17915704

8 ASSESS FOR NUTRIENT DEFICIENCIES

Summary

The main point that we want you to take away from this chapter is that if you are deficient in any one of a number of key nutrients, it is likely that this will be preventing you from getting healthy and may be one of the underlying causes of why you have cancer. In addition to reading this chapter you may want to have an assessment done by someone qualified in nutritional medicine.

PROTEIN

Protein is the one essential nutrient that you must always check that you are getting in adequate quantities. Protein gives your body the ingredients needed for every structural and functional aspect of your body. With protein you build your immune system, your gastrointestinal system, heart muscle, lungs, skeletal muscle and functional things like enzymes, etc, etc. Eggs, fish, legumes and lean meats are the best sources of protein. If you are a vegetarian then you will need to make sure that your vegetable and grain combinations are working to give you the full range of protein needed for good health.

Now let's look at why you may be deficient in protein without even knowing it.

Your pancreas makes digestive enzymes from protein and these enzymes are sent down into your small intestine as part of the process of breaking up proteins and helping them to pass through the lining of the gastrointestinal system. Many people get so low in protein that they don't make enough of these digestive enzymes to facilitate the process of digesting and absorbing protein. So even though your diet may be brought back to be adequate in protein you may not be actually receiving these proteins where they are needed. Digestive enzymes are readily available from pharmacies and health practitioners so you may need to take some of these with food for a short time to break the cycle.

If you are taking a drug that is a H2 blocker or proton pump inhibitor you are taking a class of drug whose main action is a pronounced and long-lasting reduction of gastric acid production. Gastric acid is produced in cells around the stomach and is needed in the stomach to break down proteins before they leave the stomach so that they will be in a form ready for the action of the digestive enzymes in the small intestine. Research[1] has also shown that the gastric acid barrier not only controls the colonization and growth of oropharyngeal bacteria, but also regulates the population and composition of lower intestinal microflora. Thus lower gastric acid can result in other digestive complications. So if you are taking one of these drugs it is likely that your gastric acid level will be too low to enable you to break down and absorb all the protein that you need and you will be having other gastrointestinal problems. Now H2 blockers and proton pump inhibitors are normally prescribed by medical practitioners to prevent acidic reflux into your oesophagus which is a dangerous condition and can lead to cancer. The primary cause of oesophageal reflux is obesity, i.e. your fat gut putting so much pressure on your stomach that acid is forced back up your oesophagus. See our book titled 'FEAR Made You Fat & Not Calories' to work on getting rid of that fat gut. As you get rid of the fat gut you can gradually withdraw from the H2 blockers and proton pump inhibitors with your doctor monitoring your progress to make sure you are not at any risk. If you have another cause of oesophageal reflux you may need further assistance to withdraw from this class of drug. During the withdrawal process you may need to use protein powders and other protein sources that need less gastric acid to break them down.

The way your body responds to stress could be another reason why you are not absorbing enough protein from your diet. The fight-or-flight response (short-term stress) goes something like this: When a villager in Africa sees a lion charging at him, for example, the brain sends a signal to the adrenal gland to create hormones called cortisol and adrenaline, which have many different effects on the body, from increasing heart rate and breathing to dilating blood vessels so that blood can flow quickly to the muscles in the legs and slowing digestion. Besides helping our villager run away, this type of acute stress also boosts the immune response for three to five days (presumably to help him heal after the lion takes a swipe at him). Health problems start to arise when you are continuing to respond to stress over an extended period of time as is the case in our modern society with anything from traffic noise to people complaining, having the potential to stimulate the stress response. We know that high cortisol levels have an effect on the digestion process, with a possible reduction in the amount of protein absorbed from a meal but this is probably the most under-researched area in nutrition. It is likely that chronic stress creates a stop/start process with some meals working well and the protein gets through while other meals the protein absorbed is small. If you suspect that your stress response is causing a protein absorption problem for you, then the simple answer is to find a supplement containing betaine hydrochloride (i.e. the main ingredient in stomach acid) and digestive enzymes and take these with your protein meal. There are also medicines that can help modify your stress response or help you adapt to it, so these may be worth investigating as well.

There are many other reasons why you may not be getting enough protein and consistent, thorough investigation is needed to track down things like pancreatic obstruction, lack of carrier proteins for transport of amino acids across the gastrointestinal lining, drinking alcohol with meals, infection with Helicobacter pylori[2] are all risk factors for declining absorption of protein. A variety of drugs can interfere with the process of transporting amino acids through the lining of the gastrointestinal system. Autoimmune destruction of gastric parietal cells is another potential issue. So if you are still having problems with protein absorption you may need to seek out a medical practitioner who actually has enough time to track down the cause of your protein absorption problem.

VITAMIN D

While protein is the most essential of all the key nutrients, Vitamin D is the key nutrient that most people are likely to have low levels.

Most of what science knows about vitamin D and its importance in your body has been discovered since the year 2003. The wide spread campaigns against exposing your skin to sunlight were started long before scientists realised the critical importance of vitamin D to your health. Research varies on the level of vitamin D deficiency but most research suggests that it is high, with 68% to 80% of people being potentially deficient in vitamin D [3,4]. It appears that all cells and tissue in your body have vitamin D receptors[5] and they all need vitamin D for well-being. Vitamin D has been related to the regulation of large numbers of genes in your body and is involved in many of the complex metabolic processes that your body carries out daily including the rate at which you burn fat for energy. One study showed that the greater your body fat, the greater was your requirement for vitamin D to remain healthy[6].

As the body of knowledge about vitamin D grows the more we start to realise that vitamin D deficiency could easily be one of the key factors in promoting chronic diseases including cancer.

Your skin naturally produces your body's supply of vitamin D from direct exposure to bright sun with around fifteen minutes of exposure to 20% of your skin per day regarded as the minimum necessary for good health. Depending on the conditions and the skin type some people may need around an hour of sun exposure so if you are relying on sun exposure as your only source of vitamin D it is best to get some professional advice on how much exposure that you need. Current public health warnings caution against extensive midday sun exposure so it may be better to spend 20 minutes or so earlier in the day. You should have your vitamin D levels checked, particularly after the onset of winter and supplement if needed. However, some scientists believe that the form of vitamin D formed in your skin by sun exposure cannot be exactly duplicated in supplement form and so you should not rely on supplements as your only source of vitamin D.

VITAMIN K2

There are three known forms of vitamin K. K1 (Phylioquinone) is sourced from plants, K2 (Menaquinone) is from a bacterial source and K3 (Menadione) is a synthetic form of vitamin K. K3 is usually not recommended as a good source for consumption as its biochemical structure is very different to vitamin K1 and K2 and so is not likely to perform the same functions in your body. Long term use of K3 could actually be harmful and you should only use it under the supervision of a qualified practitioner.

Vitamin K is essential for blood clotting, bone mineralisation and calcium metabolism – three issues frequently found in people with chronic diseases[7,8,9.]

The best sources of vitamin K1 is broccoli, cabbage, eggs, kale, lettuce, pork, soy beans, spinach or soybean oil and bacterial synthesis in the gut.

It is important to note that K2 is produced by gut bacteria or is available in fermented foods, particularly fermented cheese and the Japanese food natto.

With healthy eating it is likely that you will gradually pick up your vitamin K1 levels, if indeed you were deficient to start with. However, vitamin K2 is another story as the dietary sources are rarely used in the Western diet. Consequently, people eating a Western diet are relying completely on their gut bacteria to produce K2. As we have seen above, it is very common for people suffering from chronic disease to have an imbalance in the gut bacteria levels which reduces the chances that vitamin K2 will be available in adequate quantities.

The body of scientific evidence about vitamin K2 is growing rapidly and some of this is listed below:

1. One research group found that dietary intake of vitamin K2 (and not K1) reduces the risk of prostate cancer[10] - men taking the highest amounts of K2 have about 50 percent less prostate cancer.
2. The Rotterdam Study[11] highlighted the importance of getting adequate amounts of K2 by showing that people who consume 45 mcg of K2 daily live seven years longer than people getting 12 mcg per day.
3. A study[12] published in September 2009 using data from the Prospect Study with 16,000 people followed for 10 years showed that each additional 10 mcg of K2 in the diet results in 9 percent fewer cardiac events.
4. Another study[13] published in August 2010 demonstrated that vitamin K2 therapy improves bone remodelling in haemodialysis patients with a low intact parathyroid hormone level.
5. Preliminary research (published in September 2010) on liver cancer cells indicates that vitamin K2 may be useful in inducing normal cell death[14]

6. German researchers have identified that dietary intake of vitamin K2 is associated with a reduced risk of both cancer occurring and of fatal cancer[15]

7. A vitamin K2 therapeutic treatment for osteoporosis is approved in Japan. Japanese researchers[16] have been able to demonstrate that fermented soybean (Natto) which is high in K2 is useful for premenopausal women in promoting bone formation. Another group of Japanese researchers[17] have carried out research on rats showing that vitamin K2 is effective in promoting the healing of severed bones.

8. A variety of other research is being conducted into vitamin K including its possible therapeutic role in non-Hodgkin lymphoma and its possible therapeutic use in brain disease.

It is quite possible that someone with cancer will have a deficiency in protein, vitamin D and vitamin K2. Correction of these deficiencies is essential to restore good health and to put your body in a position where it can manage the cancer.

CALCIUM

We always check for low calcium levels in the diet and if necessary supplement to bring back to recommended dietary levels. Low calcium levels can promote cancer by increasing the level of Parathyroid Hypertensive Factor (PHF) which signals cells to take up calcium but when chronically in excess this hormone can create excessive intracellular calcium which then stimulates cellular proliferation – one of those strange 'catch 22's' which is easily corrected when dietary calcium levels are brought back to recommended levels (by supplementation if necessary).

ZINC

Zinc deficiency can be associated with a number of cancers and it is essential that you have adequate amounts of zinc because it is involved with over 300 different enzyme systems in the body and it is involved with the action of the immune system – supplementation is only needed if there is a deficiency. Be careful to only supplement if you have a deficiency because excess zinc can be harmful in many ways.

GLUTATHIONE

Due to its many important roles, Glutathione can run low due to the actions of the cancer or the cancer therapy. If supplies are low it will be beneficial to supplement with Glutathione.

Glutathione is a particular important molecule – it is formed from glutamate, cysteine and glycine. It protects cells against oxidative damage by removing hydrogen peroxide. Glutathione is very abundant in the liver where it has many functions. In particular it conjugates with fat-soluble toxins and drug metabolites to form water-soluble products for excretion. Another role is transporting amino acids across the plasma membrane into the cytosal by the y-glutamyl cycle. Glutathione reacts with the amino acid to form the dipeptides 'y-glutamyl-amino acid' and y-cysteinyl-glycine in a reaction catalysed by y-glutamyltranspeptidase (y-GT) and y-Glutamylcylclotransferase then liberates the amino acid into the cytosal. y-GT is located on the outer surface of the plasma membrane, and after consumption of alcohol it is dislodged and appears in the plasma. This is one of the reasons why alcohol is on the 'Avoid' list when you are being treated for cancer.

FIBRE

Check that your diet has adequate fibre as this can be metabolised to butyrate in the lumen of the gut, which can help with production of enzymes needed in detoxification and can also help with the induction of apoptosis. Our healthy eating guidelines will help you build adequate amounts of fibre into your diet.

FOLIC ACID

If dietary sources of folic acid are low then it may be necessary to supplement with folic acid to ensure there is no limitation to the anticancer actions of the whole treatment program. Best dietary sources of folic acid are beans, eggs, green leafy vegetables, and lentils.

MELATONIN

Melatonin levels are often deficient in cancer patients – melatonin has a number of important roles to play in the body repair process while you are asleep – it inhibits a number of transcription factors such as Nuclear Factor Kappa B and Tumour Necrosing Factor – it simulates the immune system and reduces the effects of cachexia.

You can ask your doctor to assess your melatonin levels and find out the best way to correct the imbalance.

References

1. Kanno T, et al, 2009, Gastric acid reduction leads to an alteration in lower intestinal microflora, Biochem Biophys Res Commun, 17;381(4):666-70, PMID: 1924876

2. Adamu MA, et al, 2010, Incidence and risk factors for the development of chronic atrophic gastritis: Five year follow-up of a population-based cohort study, *International Journal of Cancer*, PMID: 20503273 [Epub ahead of print]

3. Pitman MS, et al, 2011, Vitamin D Deficiency in the Urological Population: A Single Center Analysis, *J Urol*, 2011 Aug 17[Epub ahead of print], PMID: 21855943

4. Gonzalez-Goss M, et al, 2011, Vitamin D status among adolescents in Europe: the Healthy Lifestyle in Europe by Nutrition in Adolescence study, *Br J Nutr*, Aug 17:1-10. [Epub ahead of print], PMID: 21846429

5. Makariou S, et al, 2011, Novel roles of vitamin D in disease: what is new in 2011?, Eur J Intern Med, ; 22(4):355-62, PMID: 21767752

6. Arunabh S, et al, 2003, Body fat content and 25-hydroxyvitamin D levels in healthy women, *J Clin Endocrinol Metab*, 88(1):157-61, PMID: 12519845

7. Koshiharay Y, et al, 2003, Vitamin K stimulates osteoblastogenesis and inhibits osteoclastogenesis in human bone marrow cell culture, *Journal of Endocrinology*, 176(3):339-48, PMID 12630919

8. Ishida Y, 2008, Vitamin K2, *Clinical Calcium*, 18(10):1476-82, PMID 18830045

9. Yamauchi M, et al, 2010, Relationships between undercarboxylated osteocalcin and vitamin K intakes, bone turnover, and bone mineral density in healthy women, *Clinical Nutrition*, PMID: 20332058

10. Nimptsch K, et al, 2008, Dietary intake of vitamin K and risk of prostate cancer in the Heidelberg cohort of the European Prospective Investigation into Cancer and Nutrition (EPIC-Heidelberg), *American Journal of Clinical Nutrition*, 87(4): 985-992

11. Geleijnse J, et al, 2004, Dietary Intake of Menaquinone is Associate with a Reduced Risk of Coronary Heart Disease: The Rotterdam Study, *The American Journal of Nutritional Sciences*, 134:310-3105

12. Gast GC, et al, 2009, A high menaquinone intake reduce the incidence of coronary heart disease, *Nutr Metab Cardiovasc Dis*, 19(7):504-10, PMID: 19179058
13. Ochiai M, et al, August 2010, Vitamin K(2) Alters Bone Metabolism Markers in Hemodialysis Patients with a Low Serum Parathyroid Hormone Level, *Nephron Clin Pract*, 117(1):c15-c19, PMID: 20689320
14. Li L, et al, September 2010, Induction of apoptosis in hepatocellular carcinoma Smmc-7721 cells by vitamin K(2) is associated with p53 and independent of the intrinsic apoptotic pathway, *Mol Cell Biochem*, 342(1-2): 125-31, PMID: 20449638
15. Nimptsch K, et al, May 2010, Dietary vitamin K intake in relation to cancer incidence and mortality: results from the Heidelberg cohort of the European Prospective Investigation into Cancer and Nutrition (EPIC-Heidelberg), *American Journal of Clinical Nutrition*, 91(5):1348-58, PMID: 20335553
16. Katsuyama H, et al, 2004, Promotion of bone formation by fermented soybean (Natto) intake in premenopausal women, *J Nutr Sci Vitaminol* (Tokyo), 50(2):114-20
17. Iwamoto J, et al, March 2010, Vitamin K2 promotes bone healing in a rat femoral osteotomy model with or without glucocorticoid treatment, *Calcit Tissue Int*, 86(3):234-41, PMID: 20111958

9 LOOK FOR BACTERIAL & VIRAL ISSUES

Knowledge about bacteria and viruses is incredibly important to maintaining good health.   Bacteria and viruses are frequently associated with cancer either as one of the underlying causes or as a side effect of the cancer.

A virus is a small infectious agent that can replicate only inside the living cells of organisms. Most viruses are too small to be seen directly even with a powerful microscope. The average virus is about one one-hundredth the size of the average bacterium. Viruses infect all types of organisms, from us to animals, plants and bacteria. There are about 5,000 viruses that scientists have studied in detail, but there are millions of different types. A sub-specialty of microbiology is allocated to the study of viruses – called virology.

How viruses spread - Viruses spread in many ways including:

1. plant viruses are often transmitted from plant to plant by insects that feed on sap such as aphids – so use natural pest control techniques in your garden to control insect infestation
2. animal and human viruses can be carried by blood-sucking insects – so work with your local council to eliminate mosquito breeding – particularly important in high rainfall areas
3. Influenza viruses are spread by coughing and sneezing and subsequent contact with infected areas – so keep areas used by many people constantly clean like work kitchens, toilets, photocopiers, hand rails, etc. If you have an infection be

careful not to spread it – children are the biggest spreaders of infection, so teach them about hygiene and keep them home if they have an infection

4. The norovirus and rotavirus, common causes of viral gastroenteritis, are transmitted by the faecal-oral route and are passed from person to person by contact, entering the body in food or water. This is why people preparing food must regularly wash their hands and not handle money or other potentially contaminated objects while preparing food. You have a right to expect people preparing your food to be clean – report cases of abuse to your local council and to the business owner

5. HIV is one of several viruses transmitted through sexual contact and by exposure to infected blood – so select your sexual partner(s) carefully and insist on cleanliness, use of condoms, etc – before accepting a blood transfusion check that all precautions have been taken and where possible ask for blood transfusion free medical procedures.

Bacteria

Bacteria are a large group of single-celled, prokaryote microorganisms. Typically a few micrometres in length, bacteria have a wide range of shapes, ranging from spheres to rods and spirals. Bacteria are found everywhere on earth from water to deep in the Earth's crust, as well as in organic matter and the live bodies of plants and animals. Bacteria are prolific - there are roughly 40 million bacterial cells in a gram of soil and a million bacterial cells in a millilitre of fresh water. Bacteria have many functions and are vital in recycling nutrients within soil. Scientist think they have identified about half the bacteria species on Earth. Some bacteria are used to make cheese and yogurt and others are used to quicken up processes in sewerage treatment. In humans bacteria exist mainly in the skin and in the gut flora and because of their small size it is estimated that there are significantly more bacterial cells in our body than there are human cells. The vast majority of the bacteria in the body are rendered harmless by the protective effects of the immune system and some bacteria play a beneficial role. There are, of course, a number of bacteria that are pathogenic and cause infectious disease (cholera, syphilis, anthrax, leprosy, bubonic plague – to name a few). The most common fatal bacterial diseases are respiratory infections and this is why we need to maintain our lung tissue in good health, so that our immune system can respond adequately to bacteria – so we need to avoid cigarette smoke and other airborne pollutants that can reduce our lung capacity.

Building Your Body's Defences Against Viruses and Bacteria

The whole health improvement process we have outlined in this book is designed to build your defences against all pathogens, including viruses and bacteria. Our modern society is quite capable of creating a high stress internal biochemical environment in our bodies, with cortisol being one of the dominant hormones in this environment. Cortisol can effectively take over management of our immune defences and weaken our ability to use white cells and other processes to control the number and type of bacteria. The health improvement program is designed to help stress management, reduce cortisol level and stimulate our other defence mechanisms – thus giving us the ability to keep bacteria levels under control.

However, sometimes we need additional support where for some reason our defences have been by-passed. One of the ways to improve your protection against viruses and bacteria is to use mushroom and garlic, or their extracts, that have been shown by research to have some positive benefits. For acute bacterial infections, particularly respiratory infections, these can support an appropriately designed course of antibiotic drugs.

Mushrooms comprise a vast and yet largely untapped source of powerful compounds with a wide range of medicinal actions. Modern medicine has focused on the compounds which are modulators of tumour cell growth and the use of mushroom extracts are gradually being built into cancer treatment programs around the world.

The actions that have been demonstrated for different mushroom extracts include antibacterial, anti-candida, anti-inflammatory, antioxidant, anti-tumour, antiviral, blood pressure control, blood sugar control, some cardiovascular benefits, cholesterol modulation, immune stimulation, and a general tonic effect.

In regard to the antiviral actions of mushrooms there is a variety of research including the following:

- In 1999 researchers from the University of Wisconsin Medical School were able to demonstrate that a protein from the Gypsy mushroom had antiviral activity against a number of viruses including herpes simplex, varicella zoster virus, influenza A virus, and respiratory syncytial virus[1].

- Researchers at Bastyr University have shown the anti-malaria activity of Turkey tails mushroom (a mushroom traditionally used in Asian medicine, scientific name is Trametes versicolour and formerly called coriolus versicolour)[2]
- In 2009 researchers from Colorado State University were able to demonstrate that an extract from Shitake mushrooms enhanced the host protection against West Nile virus[3]
- A number of researchers have looked at Reiishi mushrooms and found positive antiviral activities [4,5]
- A number of Chinese researchers have focused on the antiviral properties of medicinal mushrooms including the Zhu ling mushroom [6,7]

Based on the traditional use of mushrooms as protection against viruses, and also the growing body of research supporting specific mushroom extracts, we have been trialing a broad spectrum mushroom extract in conjunction with other aspects of health improvement with clients suffering the effects of various viruses. The results to date have been very positive.

Garlic - In test tube studies, garlic has been found to have antibacterial, antiviral, and antifungal activity but there is little scientific evidence supporting these actions in humans. Garlic has been used as a medicine for thousands of years and was even mentioned in the bible. In a program to build the body's defence against viruses we will almost always include garlic because of its many benefits but never relying on it as a sole source of therapeutic action. You need to be careful in developing any program as some people suffer from garlic allergies but this is usually well known by the client as they are also likely to be sensitive to many plants in the lily family (Liliaceae), including onions, garlic, chives, leeks, shallots, garden lilies, ginger, and bananas

Like many other things available to us from nature, mushrooms and garlic were never intended to act by themselves as a single medicine and when treating a viral infection we acknowledge this by including them as one of the items in an overall treatment program that is designed to rejuvenate the body and stimulate all our defences. The results to date have been very pleasing and we believe the future outlook for defending ourselves against viruses and bacteria is very good.

References

1. Piraino F, Brandt CR, 1999, Isolation and partial characterization of an antiviral, RC-183, from the edible mushroom Rozites caperata, *Antiviral Res*, 43(2):67-78
2. Follow the link to Bastyr University - http://www.bastyr.edu/academic/botmed/coriolus_versicolor.asp
3. Wang S, et al, 2009, Oral administration of active hexose correlated compound enhances host resistance to West Nile encephalitis in mice, *Journal of Nutrition*, 139(3):598-602, PMID: 19141700
4. Lindequist U, et al, 2010, Higher fungi in traditional and modern medicine, *Med Monatsschr Pharm*, 33(2):40-8, PMID: 20184262
5. Sliva D, Cellular and physiological effects of Ganoderma lucidum (Reishi), *Mini Rev Med Chem*, 4(8):873-9, PMID: 15544548
6. Zhong Xi, et al, 1991, Effect of Polyporus umbellatus polysaccharide on function of macrophages in the peritoneal cavities of mice with liver lesions, *Institute of Chinese Materia Medica*, 11(4):225-6, 198, PMID: 1773459
7. Sun Y, Yasukawa K, 2008, New anti-inflammatory ergostane-type ecdysteroids from the sclerotium of Polyporus umbellatus, *Bioorg Med Chem Lett*, 1;18(11):3417-20, PMID: 18439824

10   MONITOR YOUR SYMPTOMS

An important issue with chronic disease is to monitor all aspects of your health as you implement the health improvement program. The following is a checklist that we use to monitor the progress of our clients. We have this checklist available on-line so that you can monitor your progress with a graph showing how you are changing on major symptoms over time (at www.perpetualrejuvenation.com) – there is a small fee involved and you also gain access to up to date information about health improvement.

We score each symptom from 1 to 10 with the following meaning:

- 10 = Never or almost never have the symptom
- 8 = Occasionally have it, effect is not severe
- 6 = Occasionally have it, effect is severe
- 3 = Frequently have it, effect is not severe
- 1 – Frequently have it, effect is severe
- The numbers between give you a bit of flexibility if you feel your symptom fits between the definitions with the lower the number the more the frequency or severity of the symptom.

Digestive Tract Symptoms

- Indigestion or abdominal discomfort/ pain
- Heartburn – episodic or recurrent
- Nausea or vomiting
- Diarrhoea – episodic or recurrent
- Constipation – episodic or recurrent

- Abdominal bloating – episodic or recurrent
- Flatulence – burping or passing gas

Appetite/ Eating behaviour

- Loss of appetite
- Food cravings
- Binge eating/ drinking or compulsive eating
- Rapid weight gain

Head

- Faintness or light headedness
- Headaches
- Dizziness or vertigo
- Insomnia or sleep disturbance

Ears

- Ears are itchy
- Earache or ear infection
- Ringing or buzzing in ears
- Hearing loss or blocked ears

Eyes

- Bags or dark circles under eyes
- Watery or itchy eyes
- Swollen, reddened or sticky eyelids
- Blurred or tunnel vision or visual disturbances (does not include near of fat-sightedness)

Nose

- Dripping from nose or excessive mucus production
- Stuffy nose or nasal discharge
- Sinus congestion or sinus infection
- Hay fever or sneezing attacks

Mouth/Throat

- Sore throat, hoarseness, loss of voice
- Chronic coughing or clearing of throat
- Frequent gagging or difficulty swallowing
- Swollen or discoloured tongue, gums, lips
- Mouth ulcers or sore gums
- Grinding teeth at night

Lungs

- Chest congestion or productive chest cough
- Shortness of breath or difficulty breathing
- Recurrent or chronic bronchitis
- Asthma – wheezing or coughing spasms

Heart

- Irregular of skipped heartbeat
- Rapid or pounding heartbeat
- Chest pain

Skin

- Acne
- Hives, rashes or allergy reaction
- Dry skin
- Hair loss
- Flushing or hot flushes
- Excessive sweating
- Psoriasis

Joints/muscles

- Feeling or weakness or tiredness
- Pain or aches in muscles
- Pain or aches in the joints or arthritis
- Stiffness or limitation of movement

Energy/Activity

- Fatigue, sluggishness or lethargy
- Apathy or loss of motivation
- Hyperactivity or restlessness

Mind/ Cognition

- Learning difficulties
- Poor memory
- Confusion, poor comprehension
- Poor concentration
- Poor physical coordination
- Difficulty in making decisions
- Stuttering or stammering or slurred speech

Emotions/Feelings

- Mood swings
- Anxiety, fear or nervousness
- Anger, irritability or aggressiveness
- Depression

General Signs & Symptoms

- Recent illness or recurrent illness
- Any reproductive system issues
- Underweight or rapid weight loss
- Fluid or water retention
- Frequent or urgent urination
- Genital itch or discharge

As you implement your health improvement program you can complete the checklist weekly or every second week and then check how you are progressing. After about 2 months of implementing the health improvement program you should have a pretty good idea from the checklist which symptoms are improving and which symptoms seem to be blocking your progress. Continue monitoring as you complete the other steps.

11 KEY NATURAL SUPPLEMENTS FOR ALL PEOPLE WITH CANCER

Our work with cancer patients plus our research in this area indicates that the following key nutrients are likely to be needed by anyone with cancer.

1. **Protein absorption supplements** – in previous chapters we have explained the things that block protein absorption. Invariably one of the issues will apply to a cancer patient and so we often recommend a supplement containing at least betaine hydrochloride and pepsin to assist with the breakdown of proteins in the stomach.

2. **Digestive Enzymes (Proteolytic enzymes)**[1-20] – these are enzymes made in the pancreas for digestion and also bromelain (found in pineapples) – all cancer patients (with the exception of pancreatic cancer patients[6]) will probably benefit by taking these with meals to improve nutrient absorption. In some situations it is possible that these enzymes can also assist to break up a tumour and there are reported cases of success and also reported cases of failure – when taken for this purpose, they are taken between meals with the objective of maximising the number that can be transferred to the site of the tumour. However, their use must be managed by a qualified and experienced practitioner and they should not be used instead of surgery or

chemotherapy or radiation therapy – the best that can happen with these is that the tumour will start to break up and be transported to your liver for breakdown into water soluble molecules and elimination from your body. Your liver needs to be in pristine working order and, even then, it can only cope with a small amount of cancer cells at a time, so it is extremely important that you do not overdose on digestive enzymes and try for a steady removal of the tumour. Chemotherapy, radiation therapy and, or surgery are likely to get better results than digestive enzymes so do not rely on these as your only form of treatment. Digestive enzymes may conflict with some medical treatments so discuss them with your doctor before starting on them. If you are being treated with surgery, chemotherapy or radiation therapy it is highly unlikely that you will want to use digestive enzymes to move the tumour to your liver so they should be avoided during treatment.

3. **Fish Oils**[21-29] – you need the best quality which have well balanced amounts of EPA/DHA and are enteric coated capsules so that they do not open until they reach the small intestine. Take three times per day at the maximum dose that your practitioner recommends – these will help reduce the systemic inflammation as well as the inflammation at the site of the tumour. You need to check with your doctor whether fish oils will conflict with any of the drugs that you are taking. If you are taking blood thinning drugs discuss with your doctor the possibility of dropping the dose of the blood thinners as you gradually increase the dose of the fish oils.

4. **CoEnzymeQ10** [30-38]– this has the potential to reduce tumour growth, stimulate the immune system and improve cellular energetics and so is a strong candidate to include in any cancer treatment unless it has negative interactions with the drugs being taken.

We recommend that you read the references and have copies available so that you are well prepared for discussions with your medical practitioner.

References

Digestive Enzymes

1. Novak JF, Trnka F, 2005, Proenzyme therapy of cancer, *Anticancer Res*, 25(2A):1157-77, PMID: 15868959

2. Elzer KL, et al, 2008, Differential effects of serine proteases on the migration of normal and tumor cells: implications for tumor microenvironment, *Integr Cancer Ther*, 7(4):282-94, PMID: 19116224

3. Del Rosso M, 2002, Multiple pathways of cell invasion are regulated by multiple families of serine proteases, *Clin Exp Metastasis*, 19(3):193-207, PMID: 12067200

4. Wald M, et al, 1998, Polyenzyme preparation Wobe-Mugos inhibits growth of solid tumors and development of experimental metastases in mice, *Life Sci*, 62(3):PL43-8, PMID: 9488106

5. Wald M, 2001, Mixture of trypsin, chymotrypsin and papain reduces formation of metastases and extends survival time of C57Bl6 mice with syngeneic melanoma B16, *Cancer Chemother Pharmacol*, 47 Suppl:S16-22, PMID: 11561867

6. Chabot JA, 2010, Pancreatic proteolytic enzyme therapy compared with gemcitabine-based chemotherapy for the treatment of pancreatic cancer, *J Clin Oncol*, 28(12):2058-63, PMID: 19687327

7. Holme TC, 1990, Cancer cell structure: actin changes in tumour cells--possible mechanisms for malignant tumour formation, *Eur J Surg Oncol*, 16(2):161-9, PMID: 2182342

8. Holme TC, et al, 1987, Actin in B16 melanoma cells of differing metastatic potential. Effects of trypsin and serum, *Exp Cell Res*, 169(2):442-52, PMID: 3549335

9. Beuth J, 2008, Proteolytic enzyme therapy in evidence-based complementary oncology: fact or fiction? *Integr Cancer Ther*, 7(4):311-6

10. Beuth J, et al, 2001, Impact of complementary oral enzyme application on the postoperative treatment results of breast cancer patients--results of an epidemiological multicentre retrolective cohort study, *Cancer Chemother Pharmacol*, 47 Suppl:S45-54, PMID: 11561873

11. Jedinak A, Maliar T, 2005, Inhibitors of proteases as anticancer drugs, *Neoplasma*, 52(3):185-92, PMID: 15875078

12. Van Hinsbergh VW, et al, 2006, Pericellular proteases in angiogenesis and vasculogenesis, *Arterioscler Thromb Vasc Biol*, 26(4):716-28, PMID: 16469948

13. Skrzydlewska E, et al, 2005, Proteolytic-antiproteolytic balance and its regulation in carcinogenesis, *World J Gastroenterol*, 7;11(9):1251-66, PMID: 15761961

14. Uchima Y, et al, 2003, Identification of a trypsinogen activity stimulating factor produced by pancreatic cancer cells: its role in tumor invasion and metastasis, *Int J Mol Med*, 12(6):871-8, PMID: 14612960

15. Sameni M, et al, 2003, Functional imaging of proteolysis: stromal and inflammatory cells increase tumor proteolysis, *Mol Imaging*, 2(3):159-75, PMID: 14649059

16. Sloanne BF, et al, 2006, Functional imaging of tumor proteolysis, *Annu Rev Pharmacol Toxicol*, 46:301-15, PMID: 16402907

17. Kerr MA, et al, 1975, Catalysis by serine proteases and their zymogens. A study of acyl intermediates by circular dichroism, *Biochemistry*, 14(23):5088-94, PMID: 1238107

18. Kirsch M, et al, 2005, Therapy of hematogenous melanoma brain metastases with endostatin, *Clin Cancer Res*, 11(3):1259-67, PMID: 15709197

19. Rinderknecht H, et al, 1988, A possible zymogen self-destruct mechanism preventing pancreatic autodigestion, *Int J Pancreatol*, 3(1):33-44, PMID: 3162506

20. Popiela T, et al, 2001, Influence of a complementary treatment with oral enzymes on patients with colorectal cancers--an epidemiological retrolective cohort study, *Cancer Chemother Pharmacol*, 47 Suppl:S55-63, PMID: 11561874

EPA/DHA (FISH OILS)

21. Wallace JM, 2002, Nutritional and botanical modulation of the inflammatory cascade--eicosanoids, cyclooxygenases, and lipoxygenases--as an adjunct in cancer therapy, *Integr Cancer Ther*, 1(1):7-37; discussion 37, PMID: 14664746

22. Arrington JL, et al, 2001, Dietary n-3 polyunsaturated fatty acids modulate purified murine T-cell subset activation, *Clin Exp Immunol*, 125(3):499-507, PMID: 11531960

23. Gorjao R, et al, 2007, Regulation of interleukin-2 signaling by fatty acids in human lymphocytes, *J Lipid Res*, 48(9):2009-19, PMID: 17592174

24. Murphy RA, 2011, Supplementation with fish oil increases first-line chemotherapy efficacy in patients with advanced nonsmall cell lung cancer, *Cancer*, doi:10.1002/cncr.25933, PMID: 21328326

25.   Patterson RE, et al, 2011, Marine fatty acid intake is associated with breast cancer prognosis, *J Nutr*, 141(2):201-6, PMID: 21178081

26.   Mandal CC, 2010, Fish oil prevents breast cancer cell metastasis to bone, *Biochem Biophys Res Commun*, 402(4):602-7, PMID: 20971068

27.   van der Meij BS, et al, 2010, Oral nutritional supplements containing (n-3) polyunsaturated fatty acids affect the nutritional status of patients with stage III non-small cell lung cancer during multimodality treatment, *J Nutr*, 140(10):1774-80, PMID: 20739445

28.   Brown I, et al, 2010, Cannabinoid receptor-dependent and -independent anti-proliferative effects of omega-3 ethanolamides in androgen receptor-positive and -negative prostate cancer cell lines, *Carcinogenesis*, 31(9):1584-91, PMID: 20660502

29.   Wirtitsch M, et al, 2009, Omega-3 and omega-6 polyunsaturated fatty acids enhance arsenic trioxide efficacy in arsenic trioxide-resistant leukemic and solid tumor cells, *Oncol Res*, 18(2-3):83-94, PMID: 20066898

Coenzyme Q10

30.   Hertz N, Lister RE, 2009, Improved survival in patients with end-stage cancer treated with coenzyme Q(10) and other antioxidants: a pilot study, *J Int Med Res*, 37(6):1961-71, PMID: 20146896

31.   Chai W, et al, 2011, Plasma coenzyme q10 levels and prostate cancer risk: the multiethnic cohort study, *Cancer Epidemiol Biomarkers Prev*, 20(4):708-10, PMID: 21297042

32.   Chai W, et al, 2010, Plasma coenzyme Q10 levels and postmenopausal breast cancer risk: the multiethnic cohort study, *Cancer Epidemiol Biomarkers Prev*, 19(9):2351-6, PMID: 20668119

33.   Bahar M, et al, 2010, Exogenous coenzyme Q10 modulates MMP-2 activity in MCF-7 cell line as a breast cancer cellular model, *Nutr J*, 30;9:62, PMID: 21118526

34.   Kim JM, Park E, 2010, Coenzyme Q10 attenuated DMH-induced precancerous lesions in SD rats, *J Nutr Sci Viaminol (Tokyo)*, 56(2):139-44, PMID: 20495296

35.   Reiter M, et al, 2009, Antioxidant effects of quercetin and coenzyme Q10 in mini organ cultures of human nasal mucosa cells, *Anticancer Res*, 29(1):33-9, PMID: 19331131

36.   Sachdanandam P, 2008, Antiangiogenic and hypolipidemic activity of coenzyme Q10 supplementation to breast cancer patients undergoing Tamoxifen therapy, *Biofactors*, 32(1-4):151-9, PMID: 19096111

37.   Tharappel JC, et al, 2008, Effect of antioxidant phytochemicals on the hepatic tumor promoting activity of 3,3',4,4'-tetrachlorobiphenyl (PCB-77), *Food Chem Toxicol*, 46(11):3467-74, PMID: 18796325

38.   Nicolson GL, Conklin KA, 2008, Reversing mitochondrial dysfunction, fatigue and the adverse effects of chemotherapy of metastatic disease by molecular replacement therapy, *Clin Exp Metastasis*, 25(2):161-9, PMID: 18058028

12 OTHER NATURAL SUPPLEMENTS TO ADD TO YOUR CANCER TREATMENT PROGRAM

In compiling the rest of the nutritional protocol for cancer treatment it will be necessary to assess a number of nutrients including those set out in this chapter. When considering their potential role in the treatment protocol there needs to be a double check that there are no negative interactions in your particular case. We try to keep it simple but usually find 4 to 8 from the list that are most appropriate to the condition. Even though the research supplied with each substance is impressive, please note the importance of including these substances in an overall program and not relying on any one of the following as a sole or primary treatment for cancer.

Resveratrol [1-7]

Resveratrol is a natural dietary polyphenol with plant antibiotic activity from grapes and it is present in red wine – dietary sources are too small to have any therapeutic effect – you will need a practitioner to prescribe a therapeutic dose. Studies have shown Resveratrol will support reduction in the following cancers: pancreatic[6] (possibly its most important future role is in pancreatic cancer), breast cancer, myeloma and prostate cancer – it can work as an antioxidant and as a pro-apoptotic agent and so could be useful in all cancers. However, care must be taken in using Resveratrol in conjunction with some chemotherapy agents as it may protect the cancer cell against the agent.

Vitamin B6 (Pyridoxine)[8-11]

There has been some research showing that vitamin B6 has beneficial effects in liver, cervical, endometrial, bladder and breast cancer. Vitamin B6 may also have benefits in hormone-secreting pituitary adenomas and may also inhibit colon cancer cell proliferation especially if combined with fats in the diet – so could be useful in any cancer treatment.

Selenium[12-16]

Selenium could be effective at the early stages of cancer (such as for people on a wait and watch list) to suppress tumour promotion or tumour progression. Selenium may also be useful to support the effectiveness of chemotherapy. However, it can be toxic at high doses so total intake needs to be managed carefully within dosage boundaries. Selenium has potential to be part of topical treatment in skin cancer[14]. It has been shown to be not effective as a direct agent against some cancers[16] and thus should be used as part of a well thought out combined treatment.

Quercetin[17-20]

Due to its anti-inflammatory and antioxidant activity Quercetin can support other treatments and help reduce the spread of cancer.

Curcumin[21-26]

Curcumin is another anti-inflammatory that can be extremely useful to include in any cancer treatment – particularly oral and colon cancer. The key issue is making it 'bioavailable' or allowing sufficient quantity of unchanged Curcumin to reach the systemic circulation. As scientists continue to work to improve Curcumin's bioavailability it could become useful in any treatment protocol.

Bromelain[27-29]

Bromelain has been used to support chemotherapy treatment but recent research has shown that it may have potential as a direct anti-cancer agent.

Genistein [30-35]

Genistein this has potential to be an effective support in many cancers including gastrointestinal, prostatic, ovarian, breast and haematologic cancers. However, it appears to inhibit cancer at high concentrations and has potential to activate cancers at low levels, so building body levels up to around 2-6 mg/kg of body weight is the issue and this may be difficult to achieve and monitor. So unless you have the facilities to do this then it is better not to use this molecule.

Vitamin D3 (cholecalciferol)[36-42]

We discussed vitamin D3 under the "Assess for Nutrient Deficiency" chapter. However, even if you are not deficient in vitamin D3 it may be beneficial to use as a support to your treatment program. The anti-proliferative activity of D3 has been shown in osteosarcoma, thyroid, melanoma, prostate and colon cancer and breast carcinoma cells. Vitamin D3 may inhibit the development and progression of a wide spectrum of cancers. It may, however, interact with and reduce the effectiveness of some chemotherapy drugs and so care must be taken when selecting it as part of an overall program. Recent research is showing that Vitamin D3 deficiency may be a trigger for cancer as well as being a side effect of the cancer process. The ability to measure tissue levels of Vitamin D3 is improving slowly and so it may eventually be common to supplement all cancer patients who have a proven deficiency before the chemotherapy is commenced.

Vitamin E[43-48]

Tocopheryl succinate is an effective form of vitamin E in cancer treatment and other members of the vitamin E family are also being assessed. Vitamin E has the potential to induce apoptosis in many cancer cell lines by increasing the activity of FAS and FAS ligand expression. It must also be used with caution, as when it is in oversupply in the body it can act like an oxidant with potential harm including triggering cancer.

Vitamin C [49-52]

Some studies show regression of cancer is supported by vitamin C use. However, most studies show no direct benefit of vitamin C at reducing any type of cancer. Consequently the best you can expect from vitamin C therapy is to support other therapies mainly as an antioxidant. It is useful to use in conjunction with vitamin E to eliminate any potential damaging effects of overdosing on vitamin E. It should be noted that combined therapeutic doses of vitamin E and C are not likely to be effective by themselves as a cancer treatment, while they may make a significant contribution to an overall program.

Indole-3-carbinol [53-59]

Indole-3-carbinol is an extract from cruciferous vegetable. It may have a role to play in conjunction with vitamin C in breast cancer and may also be considered in colon, prostate, cervical, myeloid and leukemic cells. Recent research indicates that Indole-3-carbinol in conjunction with other substances may be effective in preventing the development of lung cancer in current and former smokers.

Adenosine

Adenosine may be useful in leukaemia but has the potential to stimulate the growth of solid tumours – so use this with extreme caution.

Lycopene [60-64]

More research on Lycopene is coming available all the time. It has a number of potential anticancer actions. It may be involved in ROS scavenging, up regulation of detoxification, induction of gap-junctional communications, and inhibition of cell cycle progression and modulaton of signal transduction pathways. Recent research indicates it may be useful in prostate cancer and may support chemotherapy – most research shows it has potential as a support role and not as a primary treatment for cancer.

Green tea [65-70]

Green tea polyphenols (epigallocatechin gallate EGCG) may reduce tumour growth and/or metastatic capacity particularly with skin cancer, prostate cancer colon tumours and leukemic B cells. It can also act as an anti-inflammatory and may inhibit telomerase and matrix metalloproteinases 2 and 9 (note – this is why we don't recommend green tea as part of our healthy anti-aging program but it can be useful for targeted use in recovering or living with cancer). Recent research shows that green tea polyphenols such as EGCG have the potential to affect multiple biological pathways, including gene expression, growth factor-mediated pathways, the mitogen-activated protein kinase-dependent pathway, and the ubiquitin/proteasome degradation pathway. Research[70] also indicates EGCG has potential to support a program for treatment of pancreatic cancer.

Mushroom extracts [71-76]

We mentioned mushroom extracts in our chapter on 'Bacteria and Viruses'. Some cancers may have been triggered by a virus, or are in some way associated with a virus, and mushroom extracts may useful in these cancers. However, even where a virus is not suspected mushroom extracts could still be considered to support the treatment program. In regard to anticancer actions, research is progressing on various extracts from mushroom. There is research on the compounds with antitumor potential identified so far in mushrooms, including low-molecular-weight (LMW, e.g. quinones, cerebrosides, isoflavones, catechols, amines, triacylglycerols, sesquiterpenes, steroids, organic germanium and selenium) and high-molecular-weight compounds (HMW, e.g. homo and heteroglucans, glycans, glycoproteins, glycopeptides, proteoglycans, proteins and RNA-protein complexes). Another promising area of research shows that an extract from Higher basidiomycetes mushrooms may support prostate cancer treatment. A group of researchers[76] have identified that G. lucidum (a mushroom traditionally used in China) will support the treatment of colon cancer.

Garlic [77-82]

We have discussed the use of garlic under the chapter on "Bacteria and Viruses". We view garlic as a preventative rather than a treatment for cancer but further research may change our opinion. If the cancer has a viral link then garlic in combination with other anti-viral agents may be appropriate to remove the underlying stimulus for the cancer process to enable the body to get back to a position of being able to cure itself. Some recent research has shown that garlic extracts at very high doses may inhibit some tumours including gastrointestinal and cervical tumours. Other research indicates that garlic extracts in conjunction with selenium may be useful in breast cancer but at this stage further research is needed on how to achieve dosage requirements.

Beetroot [83-85]

There has been some research on a component of beetroot that indicates this extract may increase the respiration of cancer cells by up to 350% and thus normalise the interrupted respiration process. Other research indicates that even at low doses beetroot extracts can make a positive contribution to cancer treatment and so this is one treatment worth investigating when developing a treatment plan.

Limonene [86-89]

Limonene is a natural monoterpene (derived from lemons and cherries) which can be oxidised to perillic acid and may display cytostatic and pro-apoptotic effects in a number of cell lines, particularly pancreatic, gastric, mammary and liver tumours. D-limonene has also been shown to accumulate in fat tissue and display anticancer properties and so may be useful as part of a treatment of this type of tissue as well as other types of tissue.

Boswellia serrata [90-95]

Boswellic acid is an extract from the herb Bowellia serrata and may inhibit 5-lipoxygenases and TNF alpha expression. It may promote apoptosis, particularly in melanoma, colon, liver, glioma and leukaemic cancer cell lines. Recent research in regard to the Cysteine X Cysteine (CXC) chemokine receptor 4 (CXCR4), which is a key mediator of tumour metastasis, has shown that acetyl-11-keto-ß-boswellic acid (AKBA), a component of Boswellia serrata, can down regulate CXCR4 expression in pancreatic cancer cells.

Baicalein [96-100]

Baicalein is an extract of Scutellaria baicalensis and may have relevance in preventing the spread of prostate cancer and may also have some relevance in treating lung squamous carcinoma and myeloma.

The references set out below are an important starting point for your research into whether any of the above substances are applicable to your cancer.

References

Resveratrol

1. Araujo JR, et al, 2011, Chemopreventive effect of dietary polyphenols in colorectal cancer cell lines, *Nutr Res*, 31(2):77-87, PMID: 21419311
2. Niu XF, et al, 2011, Resveratrol protects leukemic cells against cytotoxicity induced by proteasome inhibitors via induction of FOXO1 and p27Kip1, *BMC Cancer*, 19;11:99, PMID: 21418583
3. Bhattacharva S, et al, 2011, Resveratrol modulates the malignant properties of cutaneous melanoma through changes in the activation and attenuation of the antiapoptotic protooncogenic

protein Akt/PKB, *Melanoma Res*, [Epub ahead of print], PMID: 21407133

4. Castino R, et al, 2011, Resveratrol Reduces the Invasive Growth and Promotes the Acquisition of a Long-Lasting Differentiated Phenotype in Human Glioblastoma Cells, *J Agric Food Chem*, [Epub ahead of print], PMID: 21395220

5. Horndasch M, Culig Z, 2011, SOCS-3 antagonizes pro-apoptotic effects of TRAIL and resveratrol in prostate cancer cells, *Prostate*, doi: 10.1002/pros.21353. [Epub ahead of print], PMID: 21308719

6. Shankar S, et al, 2011, Resveratrol inhibits pancreatic cancer stem cell characteristics in human and KrasG12D transgenic mice by inhibiting pluripotency maintaining factors and epithelial-mesenchymal transition, *PLoS One*, 6(1):e16530, PMID: 21304978

7. Delmas D, et al, 2011, Resveratrol, a phytochemical inducer of multiple cell death pathways: apoptosis, autophagy and mitotic catastrophe, *Curr Med Chem*, 18(8):1100-21, PMID: 21291372

Vitamin B6 (Pyridoxine)

8. Yanaka N, et al, 2011, Vitamin B6 suppresses serine protease inhibitor 3 expression in the colon of rats and in TNF-a-stimulated HT-29 cells, *Mol Nutr Food Res*, [Epub ahead of print], PMID: 21210427

9. Garg MB, Ackland SP, 2011, Pyridoxine to protect from oxaliplatin-induced neurotoxicity without compromising antitumour effect, *Cancer Chemother Pharmacol*, 67(4):963-6, PMID: 20976600

10. Akbavram S, et al, 2011, Use of pyridoxine and pyridostigmine in children with vincristine-induced neuropathy, *Indian J Pediatr*, 77(6):681-3, PMID: 20532679

11. Ren SG, Melmed S, 2006, Pyridoxal phosphate inhibits pituitary cell proliferation and hormone secretion, *Endocrinology*, 147(8):3936-42, PMID: 16690808

Selenium

12. McCann JC, Ames BN, 2011, Adaptive dysfunction of selenoproteins from the perspective of the triage theory: why modest selenium deficiency may increase risk of diseases of aging, *FASEB J*, [Epub ahead of print], PMID: 21402715

13. Bhattacharva A, et al, 2011, Magnetic Resonance and Fluorescence-Protein Imaging of the Anti-angiogenic and Anti-tumor Efficacy of Selenium in an Orthotopic Model of Human Colon Cancer, *Anticancer Res*, 31(2):387-93, PMID: 21378316

14. Chung CY, et al, 2011, Melanoma Prevention Using Topical PBISe, *Cancer Prev Res (Phila)*, [Epub ahead of print], PMID: 21367959

15. Yang H, et al, 2011, Chemopreventive effects of early-stage and late-stage supplementation of vitamin E and selenium on esophageal carcinogenesis in rats maintained on a low vitamin E/selenium diet, *Carcinogenesis*, 32(3):381-8, PMID: 21186300

16. Lunoe K, et al, 2011, Investigation of the selenium metabolism in cancer cell lines, *Metallomics*, 3(2):162-8, PMID: 21161099

Quercetin

17. Zhang M, et al, 2011, Antioxidant properties of quercetin, *Adv Exp Med Biol*, 915:283-9, PMID: 21445799

18. Staedler D, et al, 2011, Drug combinations with quercetin: doxorubicin plus quercetin in human breast cancer cells, *Cancer Chemother Pharmacol*, [Epub ahead of print], PMID: 21400027

19. Murphy EA, et al, 2011, Quercetin's Effects on Intestinal Polyp Multiplicity and Macrophage Number in the Apc(Min/+) Mouse, *Nutr Cancer*, 2011 Mar 1:1 [Epub ahead of print], PMID: 21391122

20. Camargo CA, et al, 2011, Inhibition of tumor growth by quercetin with increase of survival and prevention of cachexia in Walker 256 tumor-bearing rats, *Biochem Biophys Res Commun*, 406(4):638-42, PMID: 21362404

Curcumin

21. Pandelidou M, et al, 2011, Preparation and characterization of lyophilised EGG PC liposomes incorporating curcumin and evaluation of its activity against colorectal cancer cell lines, *J Nanosci Nanotechnol*, 11(2):1259-66, PMID: 21456169

22. Wong TF, et al, 2011, Curcumin disrupts uterine leiomyosarcoma cells through AKT-mTOR pathway inhibition, *Gynecol Oncol*, [Epub ahead of print], PMID: 21450334

23. Chen JW, et al, 2011, Anti-proliferative and anti-metastatic effects of curcumin on oral cancer cells, *Hau Xi Kou Qiang Yi Xue Za Zhi*, 29(1):83-6, PMID: 21427908

24. Soung YH, Chung J, 2011, Curcumin inhibition of the functional interaction between integrin {alpha}6{beta}4 and the epidermal growth factor receptor, *Mol Cancer Ther*, [Epub ahead of print], PMID: 21388972

25. Vilas-Zornoza A, et al, 2011, Frequent and Simultaneous Epigenetic Inactivation of TP53 Pathway Genes in Acute

Lymphoblastic Leukemia, *PLoS One*, 6(2):e17012, PMID: 21386967

26. Subramaniam D, et al, 2011, RNA binding protein CUGBP2/CELF2 mediates curcumin-induced mitotic catastrophe of pancreatic cancer cells, *PLoS One*, 6(2):e16958, PMID: 21347286

Bromelain

27. Bhui K, et al, 2011, Bromelain inhibits nuclear factor kappa-B translocation, driving human epidermoid carcinoma A431 and melanoma A375 cells through G(2) /M arrest to apoptosis, *Mol Carcinog*, doi: 10.1002/mc.20769, PMID: 21432909
28. Bhui K, et al, 2010, Pineapple bromelain induces autophagy, facilitating apoptotic response in mammary carcinoma cells, *Biofactors*, 36(6):474-82. doi: 10.1002/biof.121, PMID: 20848558
29. Chobotova K, et al, 2010, Bromelain's activity and potential as an anti-cancer agent: Current evidence and perspectives, *Cancer Lett*, 290(2):148-56, PMID: 19700238

Genistein

30. Seo HS, et al, 2011, Induction of apoptotic cell death by phytoestrogens by up-regulating the levels of phospho-p53 and p21 in normal and malignant estrogen receptor a-negative breast cells, *Nutr Res*, 31(2):139-46, PMID: 21419318
31. Marki R, et al, 2011, Potent genistein derivatives as inhibitors of estrogen receptor alpha-positive breast cancer, *Cancer Biol Ther*, 2011 May 15;11(10). [Epub ahead of print], PMID: 21389782
32. Sampey BP, et al, 2011, Genistein effects on stromal cells determines epithelial proliferation in endometrial co-cultures, *Exp Mol Pathol*, 90(3):257-263, PMID: 21281625
33. Lattrich C, et al, 2011, Additive effects of trastuzumab and genistein on human breast cancer cells, *Anticancer Drugs*, 22(3):253-61, PMID: 21160418
34. Jha AK, et al, 2010, Reversal of Hypermethylation and Reactivation of the RARß2 Gene by Natural Compounds in Cervical Cancer Cell Lines, *Folia Biol (Praha)*, 56(5):195-200, PMID: 21138650
35. Yu X, et al, 2010, Anti-angiogenic genistein inhibits VEGF-induced endothelial cell activation by decreasing PTK activity and MAPK activation, *Med Oncol*, 2010 Dec 4. [Epub ahead of print], PMID: 21132400

Vitamin D3 (cholecalciferol)

36. Kota BP, et al, 2011, The Effect of Vitamin D3 and Ketoconazole Combination on VDR-mediated P-gp Expression and Function in Human Colon Adenocarcinoma Cells: Implications in Drug Disposition and Resistance, *Basic Clin Pharmacol Toxicol*, doi: 10.1111/j.1742-7843.2011.00693.x. [Epub ahead of print], PMID: 21382175

37. Lehen'kyi V, et al, 2011, TRPV6 determines the effect of vitamin D3 on prostate cancer cell growth, *PLoS One*, 6(2):e16856, PMID: 21347289

38. Vashi PG, et al, 2010, Impact of oral vitamin D supplementation on serum 25-hydroxyvitamin D levels in oncology, *Nutr J*, 9:60, PMID: 21092237

39. Fink M, 2011, Vitamin D deficiency is a cofactor of chemotherapy-induced mucocutaneous toxicity and dysgeusia, *J Clin Oncol*, 29(4):e81-2, PMID: 21060025

40. Edlich RF, et al, 2010, Revolutionary advances in the diagnosis of vitamin D deficiency, *J Environ Pathol Toxicol Oncol*, 29(2):85-9, PMID: 20932243

41. Pinczewski J, Slominski A, 2010, The potential role of vitamin D in the progression of benign and malignant melanocytic neoplasms, *Exp Dermatol*, 19(10):860-4, PMID: 20872994

42. Stepien T, et al, 2010, Decreased 1-25 dihydroxyvitamin D3 concentration in peripheral blood serum of patients with thyroid cancer, *Arch Med Res*, 41(3):190-4, PMID: 20682176

Vitamin E

43. Bairati I, et al, 2005, A randomized trial of antioxidant vitamins to prevent second primary cancers in head and neck cancer patients, *J Natl Cancer Inst*, 97(7):481-8, PMID: 15812073

44. Sheweita SA, Sheikh BY, 2011, Can Dietary Antioxidants Reduce the Incidence of Brain Tumors? *Curr Drug Metab*, 2011 Mar 25. [Epub ahead of print], PMID: 21434862

45. Dong LF, et al, 2011, Mitochondrial targeting of a-tocopheryl succinate enhances its proapoptotic efficacy: A new paradigm of efficient cancer therapy, *Free Radic Biol Med*, 2011 Mar 12. [Epub ahead of print], PMID: 21402148

46. Jiang Q, et al, 2011, Gamma-tocotrienol induces apoptosis and autophagy in prostate cancer cells by increasing intracellular dihydrosphingosine and dihydroceramide, *Int J Cancer*, doi: 10.1002/ijc.26054, PMID: 21400505

47. Li GX, et al, 2011, {delta}-Tocopherol Is More Active than {alpha}- or {gamma}-Tocopherol in Inhibiting Lung Tumorigenesis In Vivo, *Cancer Prev Res (Phila)*, 4(3):404-13, PMID: 21372040

48. Suhail N, et al, 2011, Effect of vitamins C and E on antioxidant status of breast-cancer patients undergoing chemotherapy, *J Clin Pharm Ther*, doi: 10.1111/j.1365-2710.2010.01237.x., PMID: 21204889

Vitamin C

49. Ong PS, et al, 2011, Differential augmentative effects of buthionine sulfoximine and ascorbic acid in As2O3-induced ovarian cancer cell death: Oxidative stress-independent and -dependent cytotoxic potentiation, *Int J Oncol*, doi: 10.3892/ijo.2011.986, PMID: 21455570

50. An SH, et al, 2011, Vitamin C increases the apoptosis via up-regulation p53 during cisplatin treatment in human colon cancer cells, *BMB Rep*, 44(3):211-6, PMID: 21429301

51. Ichim TE, et al, 2011, Intravenous ascorbic acid to prevent and treat cancer-associated sepsis? *J Transl Med*, 9:25, PMID: 21375761

52. Cabanillas F, 2010, Vitamin C and cancer: what can we conclude--1,609 patients and 33 years later? *PR Health Sci J*, 29(3):215-7, PMID: 20799507

Indole-3-carbinol

53. De Santi M, et al, 2011, The indole-3-carbinol cyclic tetrameric derivative CTet inhibits cell proliferation via overexpression of p21/CDKN1A in both estrogen receptor positive and triple negative breast cancer cell lines, *Breast Cancer Res*, 13(2):R33, PMID: 21435243

54. Dagne A, et al, 2011, Enhanced inhibition of lung adenocarcinoma by combinatorial treatment with indole-3-carbinol and silibinin in A/J mice, *Carcinogenesis*, 32(4):561-7, PMID: 21273642

55. Weng JR, et al, 2010, A novel indole-3-carbinol derivative inhibits the growth of human oral squamous cell carcinoma in vitro, *Oral Oncol*, 46(10):748-54, PMID: 20843730

56. Xu Y, et al, 2010, Indole-3-carbinol (I3C)-induced apoptosis in nasopharyngeal cancer cells through Fas/FasL and MAPK pathway, *Med Oncol*, 2010 Jul 14. [Epub ahead of print], PMID: 20628834

57. Kassie F, et al, Inhibition of lung carcinogenesis and critical cancer-related signaling pathways by N-acetyl-S-(N-2-phenethylthiocarbamoyl)-l-cysteine, indole-3-carbinol and myo-inositol, alone and in combination, *Carcinogenesis*, 31(9):1634-41, PMID: 20603442
58. Kronbak R, et al, 2010, Effect of 4-methoxyindole-3-carbinol on the proliferation of colon cancer cells in vitro, when treated alone or in combination with indole-3-carbinol, *J Agric Food Chem*, 58(14):8453-9, PMID: 20593832
59. Wu Y, et al, 2010, A novel mechanism of indole-3-carbinol effects on breast carcinogenesis involves induction of Cdc25A degradation, *Cancer Prev Res (Phila)*, 3(7):818-28, PMID: 20587702

Lycopene

60. Yang CM, et al, 2011, Growth inhibitory efficacy of lycopene and ß-carotene against androgen-independent prostate tumor cells xenografted in nude mice, *Mol Nutr Food Res*, 55(4):606-12. doi: 10.1002/mnfr.201000308, PMID: 21462328
61. Tang Y, et al, 2011, Lycopene Enhances Docetaxel's Effect in Castration-Resistant Prostate Cancer Associated with Insulin-like Growth Factor I Receptor Levels, *Neoplasia*, 13(2):108-19, PMID: 21403837
62. El-Rouby DH, 2011, Histological and immunohistochemical evaluation of the chemopreventive role of lycopene in tongue carcinogenesis induced by 4-nitroquinoline-1-oxide, *Arch Oral Biol*, 2011 Jan 7. [Epub ahead of print], PMID: 21216390
63. Ford NA, et al, 2011, Lycopene and apo-12'-lycopenal reduce cell proliferation and alter cell cycle progression in human prostate cancer cells, *Nutr Cancer*, 63(2):256-63, PMID: 21207319
64. Sahin K, et al, 2010, Lycopene and chemotherapy toxicity, *Nutr Cancer*, 62(7):988-95, PMID: 20924974

Green tea

65. Cross SE, et al, 2011, Green tea extract selectively targets nanomechanics of live metastatic cancer cells, *Nanotechnology*, 22(21):215101, PMID: 21451222
66. Chen D, et al, 2011, EGCG, green tea polyphenols and their synthetic analogs and prodrugs for human cancer prevention and treatment, *Adv Clin Chem*, 53:155-77, PMID: 21404918
67. Sing MF, et al, 2011, Epidemiological studies of the association between tea drinking and primary liver cancer: a meta-analysis, *Eur J Cancer Prev*, 20(3):157-65, PMID: 21403523

68. Liu X, et al, 2011, The Effect of Green Tea Extract and EGCG on the Signaling Network in Squamous Cell Carcinoma, *Nutr Cancer*, 2011 Mar 3:1. [Epub ahead of print], PMID: 21391127

69. Onoda C, et al, 2011, (-)-Epigallocatechin-3-gallate induces apoptosis in gastric cancer cell lines by down-regulating survivin expression, *Int J Oncol*, 38(5):1403-8. doi: 10.3892/ijo.2011.951, PMID: 21344159

70. Vu HA, et al, 2010, Green tea epigallocatechin gallate exhibits anticancer effect in human pancreatic carcinoma cells via the inhibition of both focal adhesion kinase and insulin-like growth factor-I receptor, *J Biomed Biotechnol*, 2010:290516, PMID: 21318151

Mushroom extracts

71. Dotan N, et al, 2010, The Culinary-Medicinal Mushroom Coprinus comatus as a Natural Antiandrogenic Modulator, *Integr Cancer Ther*, 2010 Dec 14. [Epub ahead of print], PMID: 21147815

72. Lu H, et al, 2011, Polysaccharide krestin is a novel TLR2 agonist that mediates inhibition of tumor growth via stimulation of CD8 T cells and NK cells, *Clin Cancer Res*, 17(1):67-76, PMID: 21068144

73. Martin KR, Brophy SK, 2010, Commonly consumed and specialty dietary mushrooms reduce cellular proliferation in MCF-7 human breast cancer cells, *Exp Biol Med (Maywood)*, 235(11):1306-14, PMID: 20921274

74. Vaz JA, et al, 2010, Wild mushrooms Clitocybe alexandri and Lepista inversa: in vitro antioxidant activity and growth inhibition of human tumour cell lines, *Food Chem Toxicol*, 48(10):2881-4, PMID: 20647028

75. Chung MJ, et al, 2010, Anticancer activity of subfractions containing pure compounds of Chaga mushroom (Inonotus obliquus) extract in human cancer cells and in Balbc/c mice bearing Sarcoma-180 cells, *Nutr Res Pract*, 4(3):177-82, PMID: 20607061

76. Thyagarajan A, et al, 2010, Triterpenes from Ganoderma Lucidum induce autophagy in colon cancer through the inhibition of p38 mitogen-activated kinase (p38 MAPK), *Nutr Cancer*, 62(5):630-40, PMID: 20574924

Garlic

77. Ghazanfari T, et al, 2011, In vitro cytotoxic effect of garlic extract on malignant and nonmalignant cell lines, *Immunopharmacol*

Immunotoxicol, 2011 Mar 23. [Epub ahead of print], PMID: 21428708

78. Wu PP, et al, 2011, Diallyl sulfide induces cell cycle arrest and apoptosis in HeLa human cervical cancer cells through the p53, caspase- and mitochondria-dependent pathways, *Int J Oncol*, doi: 10.3892/ijo.2011.973, PMID: 21424116

79. Kim SH, et al, 2011, Garlic Constituent Diallyl Trisulfide Suppresses X-Linked Inhibitor of Apoptosis Protein in Prostate Cancer Cells in Culture and In Vivo, *Cancer Prev Res (Phila)*, 2011 Mar 16. [Epub ahead of print], PMID: 21411500

80. Tsubura A, et al, 2011, Anticancer Effects of Garlic and Garlic-derived Compounds for Breast Cancer Control, *Anticancer Agents Med Chem*, [Epub ahead of print], PMID: 21269259

81. Cerella C, et al, 2011, Chemical Properties and Mechanisms Determining the Anti-Cancer Action of Garlic-Derived Organic Sulfur Compounds, *Anticancer Agents Med Chem*, 2011 Jan 26. [Epub ahead of print], PMID: 21269260

82. Padilla-Camberos E, et al, 2010, Antitumoral Activity of Allicin in Murine Lymphoma L5178Y, *Asian Pac J Cancer Prev*, 11(5):1241-4, PMID: 21198270

Beetroot

83. Kapadia GJ, et al, 2011, Cytotoxic Effect of the Red Beetroot (Beta Vulgaris L.) Extract Compared to Doxorubicin (Adriamycin) in the Human Prostate (PC-3) and Breast (MCF-7) Cancer Cell Lines, *Anticancer Agents Med Chem*, 2011 Mar 10. [Epub ahead of print], PMID: 21434853

84. Lechner JF, et al, 2010, Drinking water with red beetroot food color antagonizes esophageal carcinogenesis in N-nitrosomethylbenzylamine-treated rats, *J Med Food*, 13(3):733-9, PMID: 20438319

85. Kapadia GJ, et al, 2003, Chemoprevention of DMBA-induced UV-B promoted, NOR-1-induced TPA promoted skin carcinogenesis, and DEN-induced phenobarbital promoted liver tumors in mice by extract of beetroot, *Pharmacol Res*, 47(2):141-8, PMID: 12543062

Limonene

86. Miller JA, et al, 2010, Adipose tissue accumulation of d-limonene with the consumption of a lemonade preparation rich in d-limonene content, *Nutr Cancer*, 62(6):783-8, PMID: 20661827

87. Manuele MG, et al, 2010, Limonene exerts antiproliferative effects and increases nitric oxide levels on a lymphoma cell line by dual mechanism of the ERK pathway: relationship with oxidative stress, *Cancer Invest*, 28(2):135-45, PMID: 19968502

88. Rabi T, Bishayee A, 2009, d -Limonene sensitizes docetaxel-induced cytotoxicity in human prostate cancer cells: Generation of reactive oxygen species and induction of apoptosis, *J Carcinog*, 8:9, PMID: 19465777

89. Zhao Y, et al, 2009, siRNA-targeted COL8A1 inhibits proliferation, reduces invasion and enhances sensitivity to D-limonence treatment in hepatocarcinoma cells, *IUBMB Life*, 61(1):74-9, PMID: 19109829

Boswellic acid

90. Park B, et al, 2011, Acetyl-11-keto-ß-boswellic acid suppresses invasion of pancreatic cancer cells through the downregulation of CXCR4 chemokine receptor expression, *Int J Cancer*, doi: 10.1002/ijc.25966, PMID: 21448932

91. Khan, S, et al, 2011, A cyano analogue of boswellic acid induces crosstalk between p53/PUMA/Bax and telomerase that stages the human papillomavirus type 18 positive HeLa cells to apoptotic death, *Eur J Pharmacol*, 2011 Apr 1. [Epub ahead of print], PMID: 21440536

92. Chashoo G, et al, 2011, A propionyloxy derivative of 11-keto-ß-boswellic acid induces apoptosis in HL-60 cells mediated through topoisomerase I & II inhibition, *Chem Biol Interact*, 189(1-2):60-71, PMID: 21056033

93. Liu JJ, Duan RD, 2009, LY294002 enhances boswellic acid-induced apoptosis in colon cancer cells, *Anticancer Res*, 29(8):2987-91, PMID: 19661305

94. Pang X, et al, 2009, Acetyl-11-keto-beta-boswellic acid inhibits prostate tumor growth by suppressing vascular endothelial growth factor receptor 2-mediated angiogenesis, *Cancer Res*, 69(14):5893-900, PMID: 19567671

95. Kunnumakkara AB, et al, 2009, Boswellic acid blocks signal transducers and activators of transcription 3 signaling, proliferation, and survival of multiple myeloma via the protein tyrosine phosphatase SHP-1, *Mol Cancer Res*, 7(1):118-28, PMID: 19147543

Baicalein

96. Gao J, et al, 2011, The ethanol extract of Scutellaria baicalensis and it active compounds induce cell cycle arrest and apoptosis including upregulation of p53 and Bax in human lung cancer cells, *Toxicol App Pharmacol*, 254(3):221-8, PMID: 21457722

97. Naveenkumar C, et al, 2011, Potent antitumor and antineoplastic efficacy of baicalein on benzo(a)pyrene-induced experimental pulmonary tumorigenesis, *Fundam Clin Pharmacol*, doi: 10.1111/j.1472-8206.2010.00910.x, PMID: 21323996

98. Kong D, et al, 2010, Discovery of phosphatidylinositol 3-kinase inhibitory compounds from the Screening Committee of Anticancer Drugs (SCADS) library, *Biol Pharm Bull*, 33(9):1600-4, PMID: 20823581

99. Wang L, et al, 2010, Flavonoid baicalein suppresses adhesion, migration and invasion of MDA-MB-231 human breast cancer cells, *Cancer Lett*, 297(1):42-8, PMID: 20580866

100.   Jiang RH, et al, 2010, Opposite expression of securin and ?-H2AX regulates baicalein-induced cancer cell death, *J Cell Biochem*, 111(2):274-83, PMID: 20506293

13 LIVING WITH CANCER

We have provided a lot of detail in this book about cancer and about getting healthy. There is of course much more information available and, in fact, we have written several books in regard to different aspects of natural medicine and health improvement. Our website www.natmed4u.com provides an ongoing and current resource for anyone wanting to keep up to date with the scientific knowledge that supports health improvement. If you find the technical information too difficult to follow then seek out medical practitioners in your area who have a good knowledge of nutritional medicine and use the details in this book to ask them questions about matters that you do not fully understand.

By implementing the checklist and utilising the information provided we hope this enables you at a minimum to "live with cancer". Over time your health should continue to improve, the medical knowledge about your cancer should continue to increase and new solutions may then become available.

So stay up to date and stay healthy.

ABOUT THE AUTHORS

Ron Fisher and Caryn Wichmann are both qualified naturopathic doctors and are registered in Australia as naturopaths and nutritionists. They are the founders and principals of the Perpetual Wellbeing Clinic which is a Naturopathic and Nutritional Medicine clinic in the city of Brisbane, Australia.

Their formal qualifications are:

Ron Fisher, N.D, BHSc(Nat), GradDipBus(Acc), ATMS, CPA, FAICD

Caryn Wichmann, N.D, BHSc(Nut), BHSc(Nat), ANTA

While treating clients at the Perpetual Wellbeing Clinic, Ron & Caryn would regularly come across people with complicated health issues that could not be resolved by conventional drug treatment or by traditional natural medicines. They made a decision to devote hours of unpaid research to each one of these cases to find out what was the underlying cause and come up with solutions. The result of this work was creative solutions to health problems and a dramatic improvement in the treatment protocols that were used for all their clients.

Ron & Caryn decided to spread the results of their work more broadly by publishing several books including this book on cancer and others covering most areas of natural medicine including weight loss, gastrointestinal diseases and pregnancy and preconception protocols.

To support their treatment protocols, Ron and Caryn did extensive research to come up with the best supplements and herbal medicines that supported their treatment protocols which you can find at www.natmed4u.com

The principles that guide their work and their lives are:

- First do no harm – since Hippocrates all medical practitioners have followed this principle and we know that all those who care about people will also follow this principle,
- Negotiate better outcomes for everyone – although hard work the results are worth the effort,
- Take personal responsibility for your actions,
- Lend a helping hand, and
- Use the best available scientific knowledge to constantly improve your health.

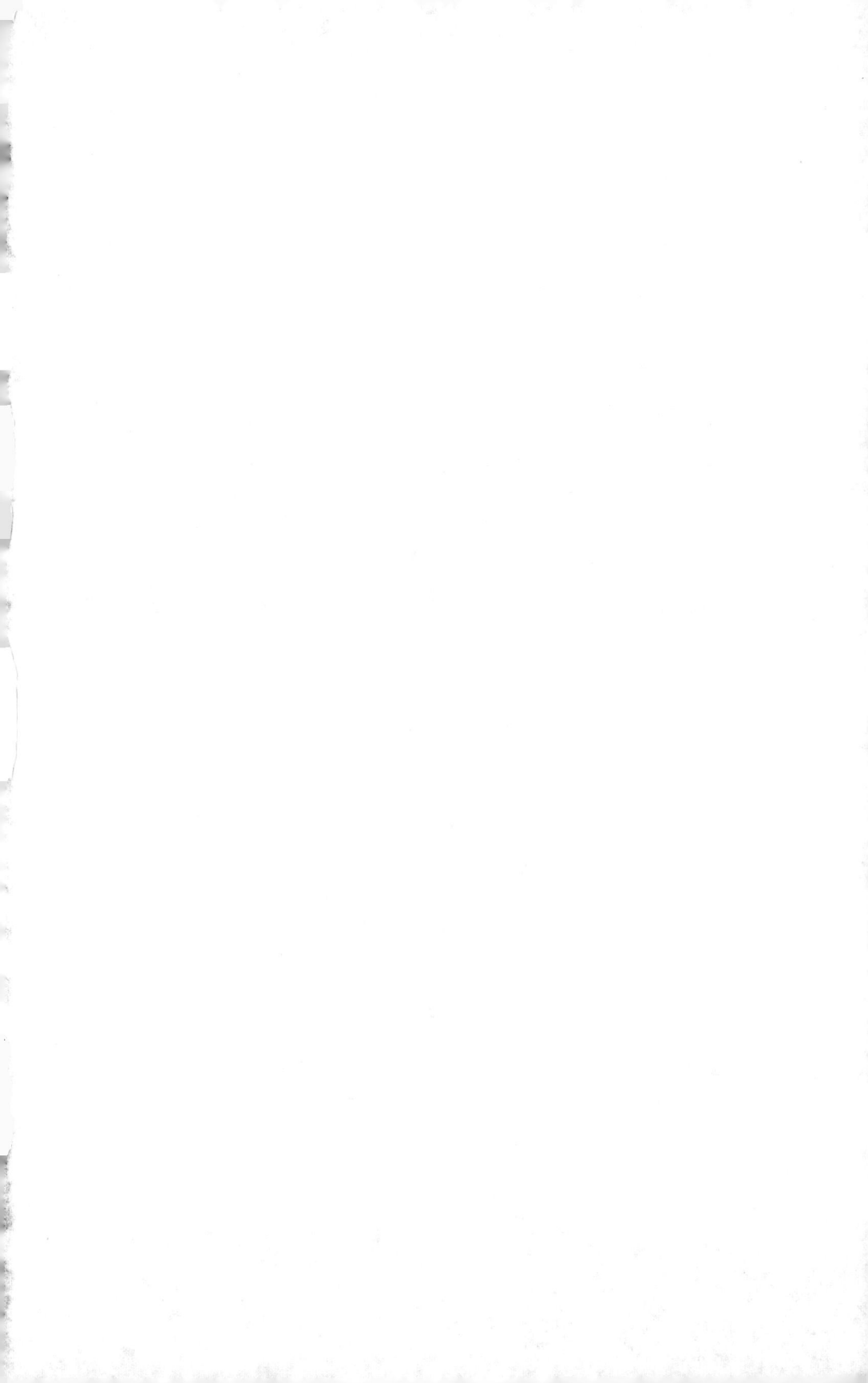

www.ingramcontent.com/pod-product-compliance
Lightning Source LLC
Chambersburg PA
CBHW060152290526
45789CB00003B/1009